LIPPINCOTT'S
REVIEW SERIES

Fluids and
Electrolytes

LIPPINCOTT'S
REVIEW SERIES

Fluids and Electrolytes

Catherine Paradiso, RN, CCRN, MSN

Clinical Nurse Specialist
Mobile Health Unit Coordinator
The Visiting Nurse Association
Home Care of Staten Island
Lake Avenue Office
Staten Island, New York

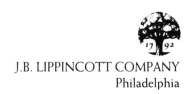

J.B. LIPPINCOTT COMPANY
Philadelphia

Executive Editor: Donna L. Hilton, RN, BSN
Editorial Assistant: Susan M. Keneally
Project Editor: Barbara Ryalls
Indexer: Ellen Murray
Design Coordinator: Doug Smock
Production Manager: Helen Ewan
Production Coordinator: Nannette Winski
Compositor: Pine Tree Composition, Inc.
Printer/Binder: R.R. Donnelley & Sons Company/Crawfordsville

6 5 4 3 2 1

Library of Congress Cataloging-in-Publication Data

Fluids and electrolytes / [edited by] Catherine Paradiso.
    p.   cm.—(Lippincott's review series)
    Includes bibliographical references and index.
    ISBN 0-397-55083-9
    1. Water-electrolyte imbalances—Outlines, syllabi, etc.   2. Water
 –electrolyte imbalances—Nursing—Outlines, syllabi, etc.   3. Water
 –electrolyte balance (Physiology)—Outlines, syllabi, etc.
 I. Paradiso, Catherine.   II. Series.
 RC630F5924   1995
 616.3'99—dc20   94-23575
                                                           CIP

⊗ This Paper Meets the Requirements of ANSI/NISO Z39.48-1992 (Permanence of Paper).

Any procedure or practice described in this book should be applied by the health care practitioner under appropriate supervision in accordance with professional standards of care used with regard to the unique circumstances that apply in each practice situation. Care has been taken to confirm the accuracy of information presented and to describe generally accepted practices. However, the authors, editors, and publisher cannot accept any responsibility for errors or omissions or for any consequences from application of the information in this book and make no warranty, express or implied, with respect to the contents of the book.

Every effort has been made to ensure drug selections and dosages are in accordance with current recommendations and practice. Because of ongoing research, changes in government regulations, and the constant flow of information on drug therapy, reactions, and interactions, the reader is cautioned to check the package insert for each drug for indications, dosages, warnings, and precautions, particularly if the drug is new or infrequently used.

REVIEWER

_____

Joanne Lavin, RN, EdD
Associate Professor
Kingsborough Community College of the City University of New York
Brooklyn, New York

Consultant Supervision and Groups
Regents Hospital
Brooklyn, New York

CONTRIBUTING AUTHORS

Angela Curty, RNC, BSN
Nurse Educator
St. Vincent's Medical Center of Richmond
Staten Island, New York
Chapter 12

Patricia Discenza, MSN, RN
Clinical Nurse Specialist
Pediatric Nurse Practitioner
Elizabeth General Hospital
Elizabeth, New Jersey

Pediatric Nurse Practitioner
Department of Adolescent Medicine
Staten Island University Hospital
Staten Island, New York
Chapter 7

Arlene T. Farren, RN, MA
Assistant Professor
Department of Nursing
College of Staten Island
City University of New York
Staten Island, New York
Chapter 11; Test Consultant

Genell Hilton, RN, MS, CCRN, CNRN
Nurse Education Specialist
Critical Care
Beth Israel Medical Center
New York, New York

Adjunct Faculty
School of Nursing
New York University
New York, New York
Chapter 14

Joanne Lavin, RN, EdD
Associate Professor
Kingsborough Community College of the City
*   University of New York*
Brooklyn, New York

Consultant Supervision and Groups
Regents Hospital
Brooklyn, New York
Test Consultant

Donna Marzano-Perrone, RNC, BSN
Nurse Educator
St. Vincent's Medical Center of Richmond
Staten Island, New York
Chapter 12

Carmen Schmidt, RNC, MSN
Nurse Education Specialist
Beth Israel Medical Center—North Division
New York, New York
Chapters 2, 3

ACKNOWLEDGMENTS

This book and its companion, *Lippincott's Review Series: Pathophysiology,* were completed through the efforts of a team of people. I would like to thank them all for the dedication, commitment, and zeal they had for these projects. Their work is appreciated beyond words.

Rose Foltz, Developmental Editor. Thank you for devoting so much of your talent, expertise, and, most of all, your time to this project. Also, thank you for your kind and gentle patience. This book was enhanced through your efforts, and it is to the enormous benefit of the readers.

Cheryl Bryant, Manuscript Preparation. Thank you so very much for your commitment, time, patience, and, most of all, *enthusiasm* for these projects. Neither book would have been possible were it not for your work that many times was done in the wee hours of the morning.

David Reuss, Artist. Thank you for sharing your talent with me and the readers of these books. The energy you gave to these projects as well as time and commitment has made this a different kind of book.

Arlene Farren, Test Consultant and Friend. Thank you for saving us in the last days before the deadline. Only a friend in the truest sense could have come through as you did.

Catherine

INTRODUCTION

Lippincott's Review Series is designed to help you in your study of the key subject areas in nursing. The series consists of six books, one in each core nursing subject area:

Medical-Surgical Nursing
Pediatric Nursing
Maternal-Newborn Nursing
Mental Health and Psychiatric Nursing
Pathophysiology
Fluids and Electrolytes

Each book contains a comprehensive outline content review, chapter study questions and answer keys with rationales for correct and incorrect responses, and a comprehensive examination and answer key with rationales for correct and incorrect responses.

Lippincott's Review Series was planned and developed in response to your requests for outline review books that address each major subject area and also contain a self-test mechanism. These books meet the need for comprehensive subject review books that will also assist you in identifying your strong and weak areas of knowledge. Each book is a complete source for review and self-assessment of a single core subject—all six together provide an excellent comprehensive review of entry-level nursing.

Each book is all-inclusive of the content addressed in major textbooks. The content outline review uses a consistent nursing process format throughout and addresses nursing care for well and ill clients. Also included are such necessary additional topics as developmental and life-cycle issues, health assessment, patient teaching, and other concepts including growth and development, nutrition, pharmacology, and anatomy, physiology, and pathophysiology.

You can use the books in this series in several different ways. Overall, you can use them as subject reviews to augment general study throughout your basic nursing program and as a review to prepare for the National Council Licensure Examination (NCLEX-RN). How you use each book depends on your individual needs and preferences and on whether you review each chapter systematically or concentrate only on those chapters whose subject areas are particularly problematic or challenging. You may instead choose to use the comprehensive examination as a self-assessment opportunity to evaluate your knowledge base before you review the content outline.

Likewise, you can use the study questions for pre- or post-testing after study, followed by the comprehensive examination as a means of evaluating your knowledge and competencies of an entire subject area.

Regardless of how you use the books, one of the strengths of the series is the self-assessment opportunity it offers in addition to guidance in studying and reviewing content. The chapter study questions and comprehensive examination questions have been carefully developed to cover all topics in the outline review. Most importantly, each question is categorized according to the components of the National Council of State Boards of Nursing Licensing Examination (NCLEX).

▶ Cognitive Level: Knowledge, Comprehension, Application, or Analysis
▶ Client Need: Safe, Effective Care Environment (Safe Care); Physiological Integrity (Physiologic); Psychosocial Integrity (Psychosocial); and Health Promotion and Maintenance (Health Promotion)
▶ Phase of the Nursing Process: Assessment, Analysis (Dx), Planning, Implementation, Evaluation

For those questions not related to a client need or to a phase of the nursing process, NA (not applicable) will be used, as in questions that test knowledge of a basic science.

Unlike the NCLEX examination that tests the cumulative knowledge needed for safe practice by an entry-level nurse, these practice tests systematically evaluate the knowledge base that serves as the building block for the entire nursing educational process. In this way, you can prepare for the NCLEX examination throughout your course of study. Good study habits throughout your educational program are not only the best way to ensure on-going success, but also will prove the most beneficial way to prepare for the licensing examination.

Keep in mind that these books are not intended to replace formal learning. They cannot substitute for textbook reading, discussion with instructors, or class attendance. Every effort has been made to provide accurate and current information, but class attendance and interaction with an instructor will provide invaluable information not found in books. Used correctly, these books will help you increase understanding, improve comprehension, evaluate strengths and weaknesses in areas of knowledge, increase productive study time, and as a result help you improve your grades.

MONEY BACK GUARANTEE—Lippincott's Review Series will help you study more effectively during coursework throughout your educational program, and help you prepare for quizzes and tests, including the NCLEX exam. If you buy and use any of the six volumes in Lippincott's Review Series and fail the NCLEX exam, simply send us verification of your exam results and your copy of the review book to the address below. We will promptly send you a check for our suggested list price.

Lippincott's Review Series
J. B. Lippincott Company
227 East Washington Square
Philadelphia, PA 19106-3780

CONTENTS

LIPPINCOTT'S REVIEW SERIES

Fluids and Electrolytes

Overview of Fluids, Electrolytes, and Acid–Base Balance

I. Basic concepts

A. Introduction

1. A cell and its surrounding environment in any part of the body is primarily composed of fluid (water and solutes).

2. Interrelated processes maintain balance, or *homeostasis*, within and between the fluid inside and outside the cells.

3. Many organs are involved in maintaining homeostasis; these include:
   a. Lungs
   b. Heart
   c. Pituitary
   d. Adrenal cortex
   e. Parathyroids
   f. Kidneys
   g. Blood vessels

Paradiso, C: *Lippincott's Review Series: Fluids and Electrolytes* © 1995 J. B. Lippincott Company

4. Homeostasis is crucial to sustain life.
5. Nursing interventions related to fluid balance are designed to help patients maintain or regain homeostasis, which may be altered by disease.

B. Definitions

1. A *solvent* is a liquid that can hold another substance in a solution *(water)*.
2. A *solute* is a substance that is either dissolved or suspended in a solution.
3. *Body fluid* is a solution of water (solvent) and solutes (electrolytes and nonelectrolytes).
4. *Electrolytes* are chemical compounds that dissolve in a solution to form *ions*:
   a. *Cations* are positively charged ions.
   b. *Anions* are negatively charged ions.
5. *Nonelectrolytes* are electrically neutral solutes (examples include vitamins, creatinine, proteins, glucose, and lipids); the nonelectrolytes that play a role in maintaining fluid balance include protein and glucose.
6. *Electrolyte balance* describes the electrically neutral state of the ions dissolved in body fluids. To maintain balance, an equal number of anions and cations must be present on both sides of the cell membrane at all times.
7. A biologic *membrane* is a physical barrier enclosing a fluid space within a living organism (eg, the cell's plasma membrane is the phospholipid-protein bilayer surrounding its contents).
8. *Membrane permeability* is the degree to which a membrane allows any substance to pass freely through it.
9. *Semipermeable membranes* are selectively permeable, allowing some but not all substances to pass through them.
10. *Diffusion* describes the random kinetic motion (known as brownian motion) that causes atoms and molecules to spread out evenly within a confined space until the concentration and distribution are equal in all areas. Diffusion occurs:
    a. In solutions within completely enclosed spaces
    b. Through biologic membranes that permit passage of the atoms and molecules from one space to another
11. *Filtration* is a physical process in which fluid is pushed through a biologic membrane by unequal pressures exerted by the fluids on either side of the membrane (Fig. 1–1).
12. *Osmosis* is the net diffusion of water from one solution through a semipermeable membrane to another solution containing a lower concentration of water and a solute that cannot pass through the membrane.
13. *Acids* are substances that can yield hydrogen ions.
14. *Bases* (alkalis) are substances that can accept hydrogen ions; these are present as bicarbonate ions.

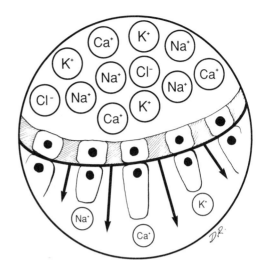

FIGURE 1–1.
Filtration. Microscopic view of glomerular filtration. Fluid (moving along with fluid is electrolytes) is pushed through small pores in the filter.

15. *Acid–base balance* refers to a state in which body fluids maintain a stable *ratio* of hydrogen ions to bicarbonate ions.
16. The hydrogen ion concentration of a solution, or its degree of acidity or alkalinity, is expressed as *pH*:
    a. Normal blood pH values are between 7.35 and 7.45.
    b. Pure water, a neutral solution, has a pH of 7.
    c. Acidic solutions have a pH below 7.
    d. Alkaline solutions have a pH above 7.
17. *Acidosis* is a condition characterized by an abnormal increase in hydrogen ions or decrease in bicarbonate ions; pH values drop below 7.35.
18. *Alkalosis* is a condition characterized by an abnormal deficit of hydrogen ions or increase in bicarbonate; pH values rise above 7.45.
19. A *buffer* is a substance that regulates pH by maintaining a stable hydrogen ion concentration.

II. Body fluids
A. Function of body fluids
1. Body fluids:
   a. Facilitate the transport of nutrients, hormones, proteins, and other molecules into cells
   b. Aid in the removal of cellular metabolic waste products
   c. Provide the medium in which cellular metabolism takes place
   d. Regulate body temperature
   e. Provide lubrication of musculoskeletal joints
   f. Act as a component in all body cavities (eg, pericardial fluid, pleural fluid, spinal fluid, peritoneal fluid).
2. Water is the principle body fluid and is essential for life.

B. Distribution of body fluids

    1. Total body water (TBW) in an adult equals approximately 60% of total body weight in kilograms (eg, in a 70-kg man, TBW would be 42 kg and would equal 35 L).

    2. Factors affecting the percent of TBW include age and the amount of lean muscle mass versus fat.

        a. Fatty tissue contains less water than muscle.

        b. Older adults tend to lose muscle mass as they age, thereby decreasing the percent of body water.

        c. Infants have a higher percentage (70% to 80%) of body weight as water; this percentage decreases as the child grows older until adult proportions are reached in the teenage years.

    3. TBW is divided among compartments, or spaces, separated by biologic membranes (Fig. 1–2); the two principle compartments are intracellular fluid (within the cell) and extracellular fluid (outside the cell; see Fig. 1–2).

        a. *Intracellular fluid* (ICF) includes the fluid in all of the body's cells; it accounts for approximately two thirds of TBW (about 23 L in a 70-kg adult). It is separated from the other compartments by the cell membrane.

        b. *Extracellular fluid* (ECF) includes interstitial fluid and intravascular fluid (plasma) and represents one third of TBW (about 12 L in a 70-kg adult). Interstitial and intravascular fluid compartments are separated by the blood vessel wall.

Total body water (TBW) = Extracellular space + Intracellular fluid space [ICF = 2/3 TBW]

Interstitial fluid space + Intravascular fluid space

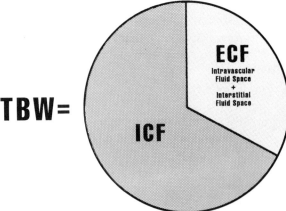

FIGURE 1–2.
Distribution of body fluids.

c. ECF is further divided into 9 L in the interstitial space and 3 L in the intravascular space.

III. Electrolytes

A. Concentration of solutes

1. All body fluid compartments contain water and solutes.
2. The concentration of solutes is in equilibrium among fluid compartments, even though the numbers and types of solutes vary between the fluid spaces.
3. Total solute concentration in body fluids is expressed in *milliosmoles* (mOsm) per liter, a measurement of the number of osmotically capable particles in a given solution.
4. *Osmolality* is a laboratory value defining solute concentration in milliosmoles per liter of solvent; it more accurately reflects the relationship between solute and solvent than the term *osmolarity*, a measurement of the number of solute particles per liter of solution.
5. Osmolarity refers to concentration and dilution:
   a. The more concentrated the solution (or the patient's serum), the higher the osmolarity.
   b. Osmolarity decreases as the solution (or serum) is diluted with water.
6. Because the osmolar concentration of body fluids is very dilute, the difference between osmolality and osmolarity values is negligible. Osmolarity is easier to measure, so it is more commonly used to express the osmotic pressure of body fluids.
7. Osmolarity normally is maintained at 270 to 300 mOsm/L within all body fluid spaces.
8. The concentration of *most* electrolytes in a body fluid is expressed in *milliequivalents* (mEq) per liter, a specific measurement of the total number of that ion per liter.

B. Electrolyte composition of body fluids

1. ICF contains water, electrolytes, proteins, nucleic acids, lipids, and polysaccharides; these cell contents are enclosed by a double-layered, semipermeable membrane.
2. ECF contains water, electrolytes, proteins, red blood cells, white blood cells, and platelets.
3. The primary body electrolytes are sodium, potassium, chloride, calcium, magnesium, phosphorus, hydrogen, and bicarbonate.
4. Major *ICF electrolytes* are potassium and magnesium.
5. Major *ECF electrolytes* are sodium and chloride.

C. Tonicity

1. Tonicity refers to the concentration of particles in solution.
2. Body fluids normally remain iso-osmolar to maintain homeostasis; such fluids are called isotonic.
3. Changes may occur in the osmolarity of the fluid in a body space

so that its solute concentration makes it either hyperosmolar or hypo-osmolar compared with other body fluids.

4. A *hypertonic* fluid has a greater relative concentration of solutes, which means that it has a higher concentration of solutes (usually sodium) in solution compared with the serum.

5. A *hypotonic* fluid has a lesser relative solute concentration, meaning that the solution is more dilute than the patient's plasma.

IV. Acid–base balance

A. Role of acid–base balance

1. Acids and bases must be balanced to maintain homeostasis in the body's fluids.

2. Homeostasis is crucial for all life processes to occur (eg, cellular metabolism, nerve and muscle conduction, and smooth muscle and cardiac muscle contraction).

3. Acid–base imbalances cause changes in the performance of certain body functions (eg, respiratory stimulation, changing electrolyte levels).

B. Respiratory regulation

1. The respiratory system can influence acid–base balance.

2. Any changes in respiratory rate, rhythm, or depth can result in changes to the balance of acids and bases.

C. Renal regulation

1. The renal system affects acid–base balance.

2. Changes in glomerular or tubular structure and function can alter the kidneys' ability to balance anions and cations.

3. The renal system will change the way it balances electrolytes to compensate for acid–base imbalances caused by other systems (eg, diabetic ketoacidosis).

Bibliography

Brunner, L., & Suddarth, D. (1988). *Textbook of medical-surgical nursing* (6th ed.). Philadelphia: J.B. Lippincott.

Guyton, A. (1991). *Textbook of medical physiology* (8th ed.). Philadelphia: W.B. Saunders.

Ignatavicius, D., & Bayne, M. (1991). *Medical-surgical nursing: A nursing process approach.* Philadelphia: W.B. Saunders.

Kinney, M., Packa, D., & Dunbar, S. (1993). *AACN's clinical reference for critical-care nursing* (3rd ed.). St. Louis: C.V. Mosby.

Kokko, J., & Tannen, R. (1990). *Fluid and electrolytes* (2nd ed.). Philadelphia: W.B. Saunders.

Metheny, N. (1992). *Fluid and electrolyte balance: Nursing considerations* (2nd ed.). Philadelphia: J.B. Lippincott.

Rose, D. (1989). *Clinical physiology of acid-base and electrolyte disorders* (3rd ed.). New York: McGraw-Hill.

STUDY QUESTIONS

1. A solute is:
   a. a liquid that can hold another substance
   b. a solution of water
   c. a substance that is either dissolved or suspended in solution
   d. a chemical compound

2. The random kinetic motion that causes atoms and molecules to spread out evenly within a confined space is known as:
   a. diffusion
   b. filtration
   c. osmosis
   d. semipermeable membrane

3. The nurse would analyze an arterial blood pH of 7.48 as indicating:
   a. acidosis
   b. alkalosis
   c. normal pH
   d. inconclusive

4. Which of the following individuals would have the highest percentage of body weight as water?
   a. elderly male
   b. infant
   c. 50-year-old obese female
   d. 45-year-old athletic male

5. Which of the following statements about osmolarity is true?
   a. Osmolarity is normally maintained between 300 and 370 mOsm/L in body fluids.
   b. Osmolarity is a measure of the amount of fluid needed to dissolve solutes.
   c. Osmolarity is a measure of the number of solute particles per liter of solution.
   d. Osmolarity is a measure of the number of electrolytes per solvent.

6. A condition characterized by a deficit of hydrogen ions is termed:
   a. acidosis
   b. alkalosis
   c. isotonic state
   d. homeostasis

7. Which of the following substances regulates pH by maintaining a stable hydrogen ion concentration?
   a. base
   b. buffer
   c. acid
   d. solute

8. When computing total body water (TBW) for a pediatric patient, the nurse is aware that:
   a. Adults have less water as a percentage of body weight than infants.
   b. Infants have less water as a percentage of body weight than adults.
   c. Adults and infants have the same amount of water as a percentage of body weight.
   d. Total body water percentage is determined by genetics.

ANSWER KEY

1. *Correct response: c*
   A solute is a substance that is either dissolved or suspended in solution.
   a and b. These responses refer to solvents.
   d. This response refers to electrolytes.
   Knowledge/Physiologic/NA

2. *Correct response: a*
   Diffusion (brownian motion) is the random kinetic motion that causes atoms and molecules to spread out evenly within a confined space.
   b. Filtration is the process by which fluids are pushed through biologic membranes.
   c. Osmosis refers to the net diffusion of water through a semipermeable membrane.
   d. This response is incorrect.
   Knowledge/Physiologic/NA

3. *Correct response: b*
   Alkalosis is a pH above 7.45.
   a. Acidosis is a pH below 7.35
   c. Normal pH range is 7.35 to 7.45.
   d. This response is incorrect.
   Comprehension/Safe Care/Assessment

4. *Correct response: b*
   Infants have the highest percentage (70% to 80%) of body weight as water.
   a and c. Elderly and obese individuals have a decreased percentage of TBW.
   d. Total body water in a 45-year-old athletic male would equal about 60% to 80% of total body weight.
   Knowledge/Physiologic/NA

5. *Correct response: c*
   Osmolarity is a measure of the number of solute particles per liter of solution.
   a. Normal range is between 270 to 300 mOsm/L.
   b. This response is incorrect.
   d. There is no measure of the number of electrolytes per solvent.
   Knowledge/Physiologic/NA

6. *Correct response: b*
   Alkalosis is a condition caused by a deficit of hydrogen ions or an excess of bicarbonate.
   a. Acidosis is an increase of hydrogen ions.
   c. Isotonic describes the number of sodium ions.
   d. Homeostasis is the state of perfect equilibrium.
   Knowledge/Physiologic/NA

7. *Correct response: b*
   A buffer is a substance that regulates pH by maintaining a stable hydrogen ion concentration.
   a and c. Acids and bases are regulated by buffers.
   d. This response is incorrect.
   Knowledge/Physiologic/NA

8. *Correct response: a*
   An infant's percentage of TBW (70% to 80%) is higher than an adult's, making infants more susceptible to complications from fluid losses such as diarrhea.
   b, c, and d. These responses are incorrect.
   Comprehension/Physiologic Integrity/Assessment

Body Fluid Balance

I. Sources of fluid intake and loss

A. Normal sources of fluid intake

1. A healthy adult ingests fluids as part of normal dietary intake.
2. Ingested fluids and water in foods account for 90% of daily fluid intake, or approximately 2500 mL.
3. Approximately 10% of daily fluid intake (about 200–300 mL) results from by-products of cellular metabolism (eg, water from oxidation).

B. Normal fluid loss

1. Daily fluid balance is maintained because the lungs, skin, gastrointestinal (GI) tract, and kidneys excrete varying amounts of water equal to the total volume ingested.
2. *Insensible* water loss is not visible or measurable and occurs through evaporation and respiration. Approximately 500 mL of water in the form of exhaled vapor is lost through respiration.
3. *Sensible* water loss is visible or measurable and occurs in the form of urine, sweat, and feces:
   a. The kidneys excrete water in urine, approximately 800 to 1500 mL/d.
   b. The skin loses approximately 500 to 600 mL of water as visible loss through perspiration and through insensible loss by evaporation; this amount can vary widely depending on

the ambient temperature and the presence of fever in an individual.

   c. Because most of the water produced by the GI tract is reabsorbed, water lost in feces accounts for only approximately 100 to 200 mL of the daily total.

4. Because daily urinary output is roughly equivalent to the amount of free fluid intake, an individual's water balance can be estimated by comparing oral liquid intake to urine output. (The other routes of water loss generally cancel out the water taken in through food and cellular metabolism.)

C. Abnormal sources of fluid intake

1. Abnormal sources of fluid intake include:
   a. Intravenous (IV) solutions
   b. Total parenteral nutrition (TPN)
   c. Blood volume replacements
   d. Colloids

2. IV solutions containing fluids and electrolytes (eg, crystalloids) are used to replace volume and correct abnormalities.

3. TPN, an IV fluid providing concentrated glucose, protein, electrolytes, trace elements, and lipids, is used for patients who are unable to take in food or fluids through the digestive tract.

4. Whole blood, packed red blood cells, or plasma are used to replace blood volume that may have been lost through disease, trauma, or surgery.

5. Colloids (eg, albumin or dextran) are used for replacement or to manipulate fluid shifts among compartments in disease states.

6. Figure 2–1 gives more information about abnormal sources of fluid intake.

D. Abnormal fluid loss

1. Abnormal fluid loss occurs secondary to:
   a. Disease-related processes
   b. Trauma
   c. Medical interventions

2. Disease-related processes that result in abnormal fluid loss include:
   a. Vomiting
   b. Diarrhea
   c. Diuresis
   d. Diaphoresis

3. Excessive fluid also can be lost if a person is breathing or perspiring at an increased rate for a prolonged time.

4. Trauma can result in whole blood loss (eg, bleeding or hemorrhage) and serum loss (eg, burns or mechanical débridement of skin).

5. Medical interventions that may cause abnormal fluid loss include:
   a. Prescribing of certain medications (eg, diuretics that in-

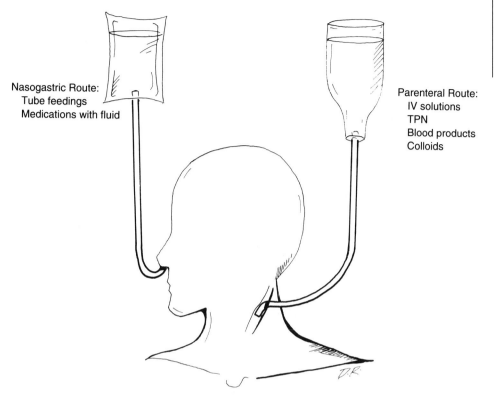

Nasogastric Route:
 Tube feedings
 Medications with fluid

Parenteral Route:
 IV solutions
 TPN
 Blood products
 Colloids

FIGURE 2–1.
Abnormal sources of fluid intake.

       crease urine output and antibiotics that have the side effect of diarrhea).

    b. Treatments such as phlebotomy (which removes blood) or nasogastric and intestinal intubation with gastrointestinal decompression through suction (which removes GI fluids and electrolytes)

    c. Surgical procedures such as small bowel resection with ileostomy, which diverts GI contents outside the body before normal fluid reabsorption occurs in the large intestine

    d. Insertion of surgical drains

   6. Figure 2–2 provides more information about abnormal fluid loss.

II. Dynamics of fluid balance

A. Passive transport

   1. Passive transport mechanisms do not involve the expenditure of cellular energy to move water (and the molecules and particles dissolved and suspended in it) back and forth across biologic membranes and between fluid spaces. These mechanisms include:

    a. Osmosis

    b. Diffusion

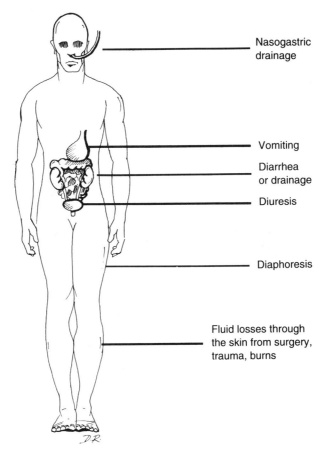

Nasogastric
drainage

Vomiting

Diarrhea
or drainage

Diuresis

Diaphoresis

Fluid losses through
the skin from surgery,
trauma, burns

FIGURE 2–2.
Abnormal routes of fluid loss.

2. Distribution of body fluid among compartments is maintained by two opposing properties exerted by solutions contained within confined spaces. These properties are:

  a. *Osmotic pressure*: Pressure exerted on a semipermeable membrane; fluids moving from an area of higher concentration to one of lower concentration until equilibrium is achieved

  b. *Hydrostatic pressure*: Pressure of a fluid mass pushing outward against the boundaries of its container (eg, the heart pumps blood, which exerts pressure on the blood vessel wall)

3. The presence of a concentration of solute (eg, sodium) draws a solvent (water) through a selectively permeable membrane when the solute cannot diffuse through the membrane. *Osmosis* occurs when there is a *pressure* gradient—a higher concentration of water in solution on one side of the membrane than the other. Fluid moves downhill.

4. In *diffusion*, the solute moves from an area of higher concentration to one of lower concentration ("downhill").

5. When the boundaries of the container are a biologic membrane, the fluid will be pushed through the membrane if there is a pressure gradient—a situation in which the hydrostatic pressure is greater in one space than in another.

6. Fluid achieves equilibrium by moving "downhill" from the space with the higher hydrostatic pressure and across the membrane to the space with the lower hydrostatic pressure. When water moves through a semipermeable membrane, smaller weight molecules (such as electrolytes) will move along with the water. Larger weight molecules (such as red blood cells, white blood cells, proteins) will remain on the other side of the membrane. This process is called *filtration*.

7. The physical processes that aid in fluid exchange at the intravascular–interstitial level are collectively called capillary dynamics, or Starling's law.

8. Capillaries are the single-cell thickness interface between the fluids in the intravascular space and the interstitial space.

9. Capillary dynamics are directly related to the hydrostatic pressure differences between the venous and arterial ends of the capillary.

10. Water, electrolytes, and cell nutrients are *pushed from* the arterial end of the capillary outward by the pumping action of the heart (hydrostatic pressure) through the capillary cell wall membrane.

11. At the same time, water, cellular waste products, and electrolytes are *pulled into* the venous end of the capillary by osmotic pressures created by the magnetic properties of plasma proteins.

12. Plasma proteins include (in order of abundance):
    a. Albumin: Maintains colloidal osmotic pressure inside the extracellular fluid (ECF) and cell wall integrity
    b. Globulins: Responsible for immune functioning
    c. Fibrinogen: Responsible for blood clotting

13. Proteins play a role in the dynamics of fluid balance by keeping fluid inside the cell (through maintenance of the normal cell membrane) and by keeping fluid in the extracellular space (through maintenance of blood vessel integrity).

14. The hydrostatic pressure generated by the pumping action of the heart is 32 mm Hg at the arterial end of the capillary, while the osmotic pressure in the interstitial space is 4 mm Hg, for a total of 36 mm Hg outward pushing pressure.

15. Within the capillary, plasma proteins (primarily albumin) maintain a stable colloidal osmotic pressure of 22 mm Hg; these plasma proteins are not permeable through the capillary cell wall, as are dissolved substances such as electrolytes.

16. The colloidal osmotic pressure combined with the tissue hydro-

static pressure of 4 mm Hg equals 26 mm Hg; the net 10 mm Hg difference (36–26 mm Hg) is the force *pushing out* fluid from the plasma volume.

17. Plasma hydrostatic pressure gradually decreases (due to less volume and greater distance from the heart) to 17 mm Hg at the venous end of the capillary, while the tissue osmotic pressure remains constant at 4 mm Hg (Fig. 2–3).

18. The total outward pushing force at the venous end of the capillary becomes only 21 mm Hg. At the same time, interstitial hydrostatic pressure, which has increased slightly to 6 mm Hg, adds to the unchanged colloidal osmotic pressure (22 mm Hg) and creates a total pressure of 28 mm Hg *pulling back* fluid into the plasma volume.

19. The net force drawing fluid into the plasma volume at the capillary venous end is 7 mm Hg (28–21 mm Hg).

20. Fluid lost from the plasma to the interstitial space (due to the greater pushing out pressure versus drawing in pressure) is returned to the circulation by the lymphatic system, maintaining normal blood volume.

21. Facilitated diffusion is a specialized type of passive transport requiring the participation of a carrier protein for some substances to cross semipermeable membranes. It is the mechanism by which glucose and most amino acids are able to diffuse into or out of cells.

B. Active transport

1. Active transport occurs when dissolved or suspended substances cross cell membranes, requiring the expenditure of cellular energy.

2. Active transport processes or "pumps" are fueled by the cellular energy released when adenosine triphosphate molecules are split (Fig. 2–4); this energy release permits "uphill" movement of substances (movement against pressure or concentration gradients).

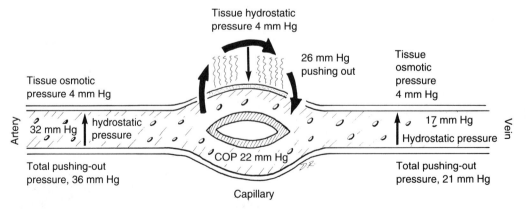

FIGURE 2–3.
Capillary dynamics illustrating pressures at arterial and venous ends.

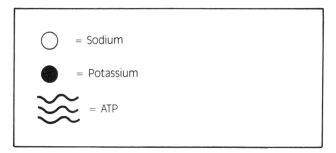

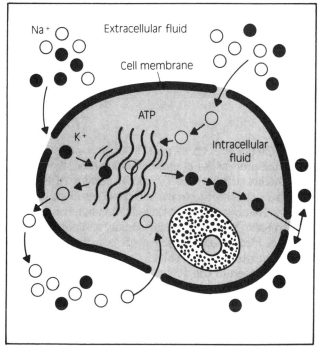

FIGURE 2–4.
Active transport. Sodium that diffuses into the cell through a
pore in the cell membrane is actively pumped out of the cell by
a carrier system (*wavy lines*). Similarly, potassium that diffuses
out of the cell is actively replaced by the carrier system.

3. Active transport can move different substances into and out of a
cell simultaneously.
4. The best known example of active transport is the *sodium-potassium pump*, in which sodium ions are pumped *into* and potassium
ions are pumped *out of* a cell during each exchange. Other electrolytes also are pumped into and out of the cell (Fig. 2–5).
5. The sodium-potassium pump plays a key role in the maintenance
of intracellular fluid (ICF) volume. The outflow of sodium ions
counterbalances the osmotic pressure exerted by the intracellular
proteins to pull excess water into cells.

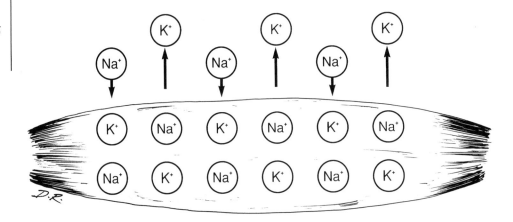

FIGURE 2–5.
Sodium-potassium pump. Sodium ions are pumped into the cell and potassium ions are pumped out of the cell.

III. Regulation of body fluids

A. Overview of systemic regulators

1. To maintain homeostasis, many body systems interact to ensure a balance of fluid intake and output and a normal distribution of body fluids among compartments.

2. The primary systemic regulators of body fluid are:
   a. Renal
   b. Endocrine
   c. Cardiovascular
   d. Gastrointestinal
   e. Pulmonary

B. Renal regulation

1. The kidneys are the major regulators of sodium and water balance in the ECF (Fig. 2–6).

2. Cells in the glomerulus secrete the enzyme renin when they sense decreased serum sodium concentration or decreased plasma volume.

3. Renin activates angiotensin I, which is then enzymatically converted to angiotensin II, a powerful vasoconstrictor.

4. Angiotensin II selectively constricts portions of the arteriole in the nephron. If serum sodium is low in the presence of increased plasma volume, glomerular filtration is increased, thus increasing urine output. If serum sodium is high with normal to low plasma volume, glomerular filtration is decreased, thus decreasing urine output.

5. Angiotensin II also causes release of the hormone aldosterone from the adrenal cortex; it acts on the distal renal tubule to cause reabsorption of sodium and water and excretion of potassium (Fig. 2–7).

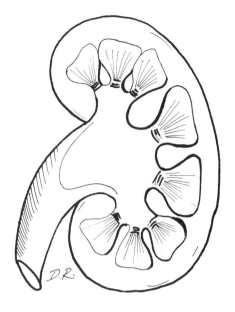

FIGURE 2–6.
The kidney. The kidney regulates body fluids and electrolytes by eliminating water and waste products, and by balancing electrolytes, acids, and bases.

C. Endocrine regulation

1. The primary regulator of water intake is the thirst center in the hypothalamus.

2. A person drinks or stops drinking water or other fluids in response to a feedback loop of signals from the thirst center and the GI tract. Decreased ICF in thirst center cells, plus decreased fullness in the gut, stimulates drinking.

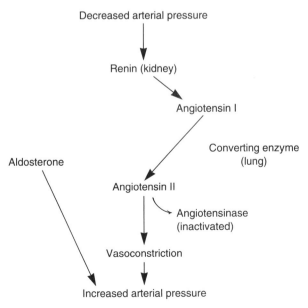

FIGURE 2–7.
Renin-angiotensin-aldosterone mechanism.

3. Osmoreceptor cells in the posterior hypothalamus respond to changes in ECF osmolarity:
   a. When ECF osmolarity increases, the pituitary gland secretes antidiuretic hormone (ADH).
   b. When ECF osmolarity decreases, ADH secretion is inhibited.
4. ADH acts on the distal renal tubules to increase their membrane permeability to water, thus increasing the rate of water reabsorption.
5. GI tract sensory receptors feed back the sensation of fullness to the hypothalamus, and under the influence of ADH, water is reabsorbed in the bowel.
6. The ICF volume in thirst center neurons increases, inhibiting the need to drink.
7. Together, the thirst feedback mechanisms and ADH function to conserve water and ensure its intake to maintain homeostasis.
8. The adrenals help control fluid and electrolyte balance through secretion of steroid hormones, mainly aldosterone.
9. The parathyroid aids in maintaining electrolyte balance through secretion of parathyroid hormone.
10. Figure 2–8 provides more information on endocrine regulation.

D. Cardiovascular regulation

1. The cardiovascular system regulates fluid volume, pressure sensors, and atrial natriuretic factor (Fig. 2–9).

Endocrine Organs and Their Function

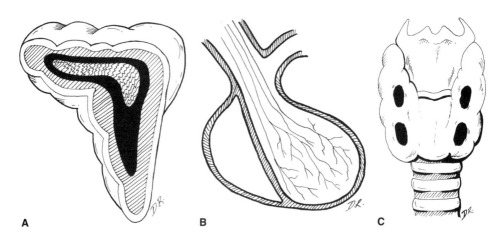

A   B   C

FIGURE 2–8.
(A) The adrenal glands. The adrenal glands help balance electrolytes by secreting steroid hormones. **(B) The pituitary gland.** The pituitary gland secretes antidiuretic hormone (ADH) that releases water in the kidney tubules. The pituitary also secretes adrenocorticotropin hormone (ACTH) that stimulates the adrenal glands. **(C) Parathyroid glands.** The parathyroid glands aid in maintaining electrolyte balance through secretion of parathyroid hormone (PTH).

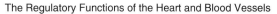

The Regulatory Functions of the Heart and Blood Vessels

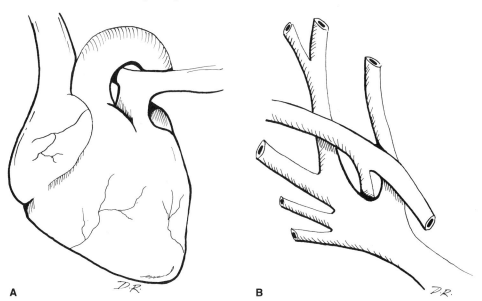

A   **B**

FIGURE 2–9.
(A) The heart. The heart regulates body fluids by propelling fluid through the body. **(B) The blood vessels.** Along with the heart, blood vessels help regulate fluid balance by vasoconstriction and vasodilation. Blood vessels contain pressure and stretch receptors that facilitate vasodilation and vasoconstriction.

2. Normal blood volume permits the heart to pump blood to the kidneys at an optimal pressure; adequate kidney perfusion allows urine to form.
3. Changes in blood volume directly affect arterial blood pressure and urinary output:
   a. Increased blood volume increases cardiac output.
   b. An increase in cardiac output causes arterial pressure to rise.
   c. Elevations in arterial pressure directly affect the kidneys, causing an increase in urine output; a corresponding decrease in blood volume completes the feedback mechanism, thus maintaining a stable blood volume in spite of variations in daily intake.
4. Arterial baroreceptors and low-pressure sensors (stretch receptors) in the larger blood vessels (eg, aorta, carotids) respond to changes in blood volume:
   a. A rise in arterial pressure causes the baroreceptors and stretch receptors to signal an inhibition of the sympathetic nervous system (SNS).
   b. Reflex SNS inhibition causes dilation of renal arterioles with a subsequent increase in urine output.

    c. Vasoconstriction or vasodilation will occur in response to arterial baroreceptor stimulation.

5. Atrial natriuretic factor (ANF) is a polypeptide hormone secreted by the cardiac atria into the blood following stretching of the atria by increased blood volume.

6. ANF signals the kidneys to decrease tubular reabsorption of sodium. As a result, urine osmolarity and output are significantly increased, reducing blood volume.

7. ANF has a short-term effect on blood volume; it appears to be counteracted by other regulatory mechanisms in chronic states of increased blood volume.

E. Gastrointestinal regulation

1. The GI tract organs digest food (breaking it down chemically into simpler, soluble substances) so that it can be absorbed by body tissues.

2. The hormonal and enzymatic processes involved in digestion, combined with passive and active transport, are the mechanisms through which the GI tract participates in fluid volume regulation (Fig. 2–10).

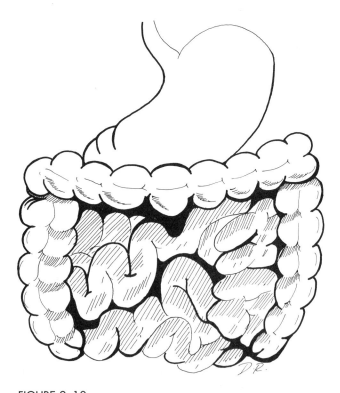

FIGURE 2–10.
Gastrointestinal organs. The stomach and intestines help balance the body's fluids and electrolytes by absorbing those that are needed and eliminating those that are not needed.

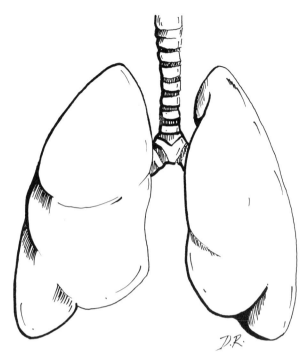

FIGURE 2–11.
The lungs. The lungs help balance body fluids since expired air is water saturated.

3. After initial gastric digestion, the fluid mixture of food, water, and GI tract secretions (a 24-hour volume of about 9 L) moves into the small intestine.
4. Approximately 85% to 95% of water absorption and most nutrient transport into the plasma volume takes place in the small intestine.
5. The colon absorbs additional water (500–1000 mL) and exchanges electrolytes before it moves the remaining waste matter toward the rectum and anus for eventual expulsion as feces.

F. Pulmonary regulation
1. The normal elimination of water through the lungs (insensible water loss) equals approximately 500 mL/d.
2. The amount of insensible water loss varies with hyperventilation and mechanical ventilation (Fig. 2–11).

Bibliography

Brunner, L., & Suddarth, D. (1988). *Textbook of medical-surgical nursing* (6th ed.). Philadelphia: J.B. Lippincott.
Guyton, A. (1991). *Textbook of medical physiology* (8th ed.). Philadelphia: W.B. Saunders.

Ignatavicius, D., & Bayne, M. (1991). *Medical-surgical nursing: A nursing process approach.* Philadelphia: W.B. Saunders.

Kinney, M., Packa, D., & Dunbar, S. (1993). *AACN's clinical reference for critical-care nursing* (3rd ed.). St. Louis: C.V. Mosby.

Kokko, J., & Tannen, R. (1990). *Fluid and electrolytes* (2nd ed.). Philadelphia: W.B. Saunders.

Metheny, N. (1992). *Fluid and electrolyte balance: Nursing considerations* (2nd ed.). Philadelphia: J.B. Lippincott.

Rose, D. (1989). *Clinical physiology of acid-base and electrolyte disorders* (3rd ed.). New York: McGraw-Hill.

Taylor, C., Lillis, C., & LeMone, P. (1993). *Fundamentals of nursing: The art and science of nursing* (2nd ed.). Philadelphia: J.B. Lippincott.

Thomson, J., McFarland, G., Hirsch, J., & Tucker, S. (1993). *Mosby's clinical nursing* (3rd ed.). St. Louis: Mosby–Year Book.

STUDY QUESTIONS

1. As part of the endocrine regulation of body fluid balance, osmoreceptor cells in the posterior hypothalamus secrete which of the following hormones when extracellular fluid (ECF) osmolarity increases?
   a. angiotensin I
   b. antidiuretic hormone (ADH)
   c. renin
   d. aldosterone

2. Which of the following body systems is *not* a primary systemic regulator of body fluids?
   a. renal system
   b. gastrointestinal system
   c. respiratory system
   d. cardiovascular system

3. Capillary dynamics are directly related to the hydrostatic pressure differences between:
   a. intracellular fluid (ICF) and extracellular fluid (ECF)
   b. venous and arterial ends of capillaries
   c. osmosis and diffusion
   d. filtration and capillaries

4. The mechanism by which glucose and most amino acids are able to diffuse into and out of cells is termed:
   a. hydrostatic pressure
   b. Starling's law
   c. facilitated diffusion
   d. colloidal osmotic pressure

5. The difference between active and passive transport involves:
   a. the type of solute
   b. pressure gradients

   c. thickness of the capillary wall
   d. expenditure of cellular energy

6. Which of the following disease states can cause excessive insensible fluid loss?
   a. vomiting
   b. diuretic therapy
   c. diarrhea
   d. fever with diaphoresis

7. The pumping action of the heart generates:
   a. hydrostatic pressure
   b. osmotic pressure
   c. oncotic pressure
   d. hypertonic pressure

8. The sodium-potassium pump plays a key role in maintaining the volume of:
   a. ECF
   b. ICF
   c. intravascular fluid
   d. interstitial fluid

9. When performing a complete fluid and electrolyte assessment, the nurse should evaluate a patient's protein levels because proteins are responsible for:
   a. anticoagulation effects
   b. vascular and cell wall integrity
   c. fluid movement outside of the cell
   d. immunosuppressive defenses

10. Which of the following hormones does *not* help balance the body's fluids?
    a. renin
    b. aldosterone
    c. parathyroid hormone (PTH)
    d. antidiuretic hormone (ADH)

ANSWER KEY

1. *Correct response: b*
ADH is secreted by the pituitary when signaled by the hypothalamus that ECF osmolarity has increased. As a result, increased water will be reabsorbed in the kidneys, thus decreasing ECF osmolarity.
a, c, and d. Angiotensin I, renin, and aldosterone are part of the renal regulation of fluid balance.
Comprehension/Physiologic/Analysis

2. *Correct response: b*
The respiratory system is not a primary systemic regulator of fluid balance.
a, c, and d. The renal, gastrointestinal, and cardiovascular systems, as well as endocrine system, are the primary systemic body fluid regulators.
Knowledge/Physiologic/Analysis

3. *Correct response: b*
Capillary dynamics are directly related to the hydrostatic pressure differences between the venous and arterial ends of capillaries and aid in fluid exchange between the intravascular and interstitial spaces.
a, c, and d. These responses are incorrect.
Knowledge/Physiologic/Analysis

4. *Correct response: c*
Facilitated diffusion is a specialized type of passive transport requiring the participation of a carrier protein for some substances to cross semipermeable membranes. It is the mechanism by which glucose and most amino acids are able to diffuse into and out of cells.
a, b, and d. These responses are incorrect.
Analysis/Physiologic/Analysis

5. *Correct response: d*
Active transport differs from passive transport in that cellular energy is required to fuel these pumps and permit substances to move against pressure gradients.
a, b, and c. These responses are incorrect.
Analysis/Physiologic/Analysis

6. *Correct response: d*
Fever with diaphoresis will cause excessive fluid loss through the skin. Since this loss is not measurable, it is an insensible fluid loss.
a, b, and c. These states will cause abnormal and excessive fluid loss, but these losses are measurable and therefore are *not* insensible.
Application/Physiologic/Assessment

7. *Correct response: a*
The pumping action of the heart is hydrostatic pressure (pressure of a fluid mass pushing outward against the boundaries of its container).
b. Osmotic pressure refers to the pressure inside the ECF and ICF.
c. This response is incorrect.
d. There is no such entity as hypertonic pressure.
Comprehension/Physiologic/Analysis

8. *Correct response: b*
The sodium-potassium pump plays a key role in the maintenance of ICF volume. The outflow of sodium ions counter balances the osmotic pressure exerted by the intracellular proteins to pull excess water into the cells.
a, c, and d. These represent the other fluid compartments in which the sodium-potassium pump has a lesser influence.
Knowledge/Physiologic/Analysis

9. *Correct response: b*
Plasma proteins, particularly albumin, maintain cell wall integrity and blood vessel integrity, keeping fluid inside the fluid compartments.
a. The plasma protein fibrinogen is responsible for blood clotting.

c. Proteins prevent fluid from moving outside of the cell.
d. The plasma protein globulin is responsible for keeping the immune system intact.

Application/Safe Care/Assessment

10. *Correct response: c*
Parathyroid hormone (PTH) does not play a role in fluid balance.

a and b. The renin-angiotensin-aldosterone mechanism plays a critical role in fluid balance.
d. Antidiuretic hormone (ADH) helps regulate fluid balance by reabsorbing water in the renal tubules.

Knowledge/Physiologic/Analysis

Alterations in Body Fluid Balance

I. Alterations in body fluid balance

A. Fluid volume deficit (FVD)

1. FVD, commonly called *hypovolemia*, is a condition in which fluid loss exceeds fluid intake.
2. FVD may be isotonic, hypotonic, or hypertonic.
3. Figure 3–1 illustrates some symptoms of FVD.

B. Fluid volume excess (FVE)

1. FVE, commonly called *hypervolemia*, is a condition in which fluid intake exceeds fluid loss.

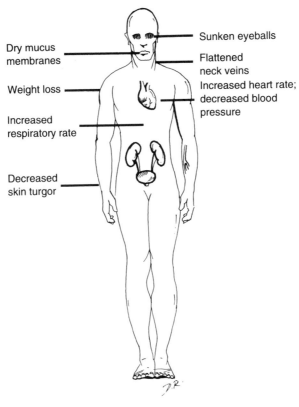

FIGURE 3–1.
Fluid volume deficit.

2. FVE may be isotonic, hypotonic, or hypertonic.
3. Figure 3–2 illustrates some symptoms of FVE.

II. Isotonic FVD

A. Description

1. Isotonic FVD is an equal decrease in ECF solute concentration (especially sodium) and water volume.
2. The ECF maintains its normal iso-osmolar state.
3. No changes are produced in the ICF volume.

B. Etiology

1. Isotonic FVD *can* result from excessive loss of iso-osmolar fluids through:
   a. GI tract (through vomiting, diarrhea, nasogastric suctioning)
   b. Kidneys (through diuresis secondary to renal disease and diuretic use)
   c. Skin (through excessive perspiration and burns)
   d. Hemorrhage

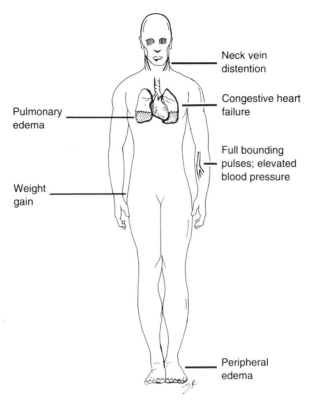

Neck vein distention

Congestive heart failure

Pulmonary edema

Full bounding pulses; elevated blood pressure

Weight gain

Peripheral edema

FIGURE 3–2.
Fluid volume excess.

2. Lack of intake of fluids and electrolytes may occur secondary to an inability to ingest orally (eg, decreased level of consciousness, sedation, nothing by mouth status).

3. Iso-osmolar fluid shifts into potential anatomic body spaces (eg, peritoneal cavity, interstitial fluid compartment) where the fluid is not readily available for exchange with the plasma volume. The interstitial space is the most common site for third spacing.

4. This phenomenon of fluid shifting into spaces other than the ECF or ICF is known as *third spacing.* It can occur secondary to:
   a. Acute bowel obstruction
   b. Infection that leads to sepsis (eg, peritonitis)
   c. Blockage of the lymphatic drainage system
   d. Liver disease (eg, cirrhosis)
   e. Poor circulation

C. **Assessment findings**
   1. Clinical manifestations of isotonic FVD may include:
      a. Acute weight loss (especially if greater than 5% of total body weight)

   b. Cardiovascular changes (eg, increased heart rate, decreased blood pressure [especially if resulting in postural hypotension], and flattened neck veins in the supine position)
   c. Increased respiratory rate
   d. Decreased hydration of the skin and mucous membranes (eg, dry tongue, "sticky" mucous membranes in the oral cavity, and decreased skin turgor)
   e. Decreased and concentrated urine output
   f. Increased hematocrit
   g. Thick and sticky respiratory secretions
   h. Sunken eyeballs

2. Symptoms of third space fluid accumulation depend on the location of the space:
   a. Ascites is fluid accumulation in the peritoneal cavity; it is marked by increased abdominal girth.
   b. Pleural effusion is fluid in the pleural space. Auscultation of the lungs in the area of the effusion reveals decreased breath sounds; the patient also may experience shortness of breath.
   c. Pericardial effusion results from fluid accumulation in the pericardial cavity; it is manifested by altered hemodynamics and muffled heart sounds.
   d. Edema in the feet (pedal) that works its way up the extremities is the most common.
   e. Anasarca is generalized third spacing that affects the whole body.
   f. Pulmonary edema is fluid accumulation in the interstitial spaces in the lung.

3. In third space fluid accumulation, weight *gain* may occur in spite of the fluid deficit in the intravascular space.

D. **Potential nursing diagnoses**
   1. Fluid Volume Deficit
   2. Altered Tissue Perfusion (the kidneys are at special risk)
   3. High Risk for Injury
   4. Ineffective Breathing Patterns
   5. Decreased Cardiac Output

E. **Interventions**
   1. Medical management involves:
      a. Replacement with isotonic fluids and electrolytes by oral or IV route
      b. IV replacement of blood, blood components, or proteins if the FVD is due to hemorrhage or fluid shift to the tissues
      c. Treatment of contributory underlying disease states (eg, prescription of medications to counteract vomiting or diarrhea)
      d. Removal of third space fluid accumulations by direct

drainage (eg, chest tube insertion to drain a pleural effusion) when indicated

   e. Mobilization of interstitial fluids (must be done with great caution because this can lead to FVE)

   2. Nursing considerations
      a. Assess cardiovascular, respiratory, and neurologic status.
      b. Assess skin turgor and hydration of mucous membranes.
      c. Monitor laboratory values (eg, hematocrit, hemoglobin, blood urea nitrogen [BUN]).
      d. Monitor intake and output; urine output should be a bare minimum of approximately 30 mL/h or about 500 to 700 mL/d.
      e. Monitor weight daily; weight loss of more than 0.5 lb/d is considered fluid loss.
      f. Provide patient teaching about medication regimen, prescribed diet and foods to avoid, signs and symptoms of the specific disorder for which the patient is at risk (eg, weight loss), and preventive measures.

F. Evaluation
   1. The patient's pulse, blood pressure, and neck veins are normal.
   2. The patient's tongue and mucous membranes are moist, and skin turgor is good.
   3. The patient's hematocrit is increased.
   4. The patient's breath sounds are clear.
   5. Perfusion of vital organs is maintained.
   6. The patient is free from injury.

III. Hypotonic FVD

A. Description
   1. Hypotonic FVD is a decrease in solute concentration with water volume remaining normal.
   2. The ECF is hypo-osmolar, and fluid shifts into the cells.

B. Etiology
   1. GI fluid loss through vomiting and diarrhea
   2. Renal loss
   3. Malnutrition
   4. Iatrogenic fluid replacement with hypotonic fluid solutions

C. Assessment findings
   1. Symptoms of hypotonic FVD are the same as for isotonic FVD (see Section II.C).
   2. Additional symptoms can include:
      a. Weakness
      b. Fatigue
      c. Muscle cramps
      d. Postural hypotension
      e. Confusion

D. **Potential nursing diagnoses (same as for isotonic FVD, see Section II.D)**

E. **Interventions**

1. Medical management involves the same treatments as for isotonic FVD (see Section II.E.1), except for fluid replacement strategies:
    a. For mild hyponatremia, replacement with oral salt and water or IV isotonic saline
    b. For severe hyponatremia, replacement with hypertonic saline solutions
    c. Replacement of potassium, if depleted
2. Nursing considerations are the same as for isotonic FVD (see Section II.E.2).

F. **Evaluation**

1. Serum sodium level returns to normal.
2. The evaluation is the same as for isotonic FVD (see Section II.F.)

IV. Hypertonic FVD

A. **Description**

1. Hypertonic FVD is a decrease in water volume without a corresponding decrease in solute concentration.
2. The ECF is hyperosmolar.
3. ICF shifts into the extracellular compartment.

B. **Etiology**

1. Osmotic diuresis or severe GI infections causing ECF volume depletion and increased sodium concentration
2. Poorly regulated nasogastric tube feedings
3. Insensible water loss during prolonged fever
4. Altered mental status in which a person is unable to access water freely; a person with an intact sensorium, normal thirst regulation, and uninhibited water access cannot usually develop a hypertonic FVD.
5. Impaired thirst regulation, possibly due to a hypothalamic lesion

C. **Assessment findings**

1. Decreased skin turgor
2. Decreased hydration of mucous membranes
3. Decreased blood pressure, increased pulse, postural hypotension
4. Increased thirst
5. Pitting edema
6. Increased respiratory rate and depth
7. Decreased peripheral pulses
8. Hyperactive deep tendon reflexes

D. **Potential nursing diagnoses**

1. High Risk for Alteration in skin integrity
2. Ineffective Breathing Pattern

E. **Interventions**
  1. Medical management involves treatment of the underlying disease process and replacement of fluid loss:
     a. For water loss, replacement with water only
     b. For sodium loss, replacement with dilute (hypotonic) saline IV
  2. Nursing considerations are the same as for isotonic FVD (see Section II.E.2).
F. **Evaluation**
  1. The patient's vital signs, skin turgor, and mucous membranes are normal.
  2. The patient breathes normally.
  3. The patient displays no signs of edema.

V. Isotonic FVE

A. **Description**
  1. Isotonic FVE is an increase in water volume and solute concentration (especially sodium) in the ECF in proportions equal to its normal iso-osmolar state.
  2. It does not involve an ICF shift.
B. **Etiology**
  1. Excessive intake of sodium and water, either orally or IV
  2. Iso-osmolar fluid retention secondary to impaired regulatory mechanisms (eg, renal dysfunction, inappropriate secretion of ADH, cardiac disease)
  3. Use of corticosteroids
  4. Chronic liver failure
C. **Assessment findings**
  1. Clinical manifestations include:
     a. Circulatory overload
     b. Interstitial edema
     c. Rapid weight gain (especially if greater than 5% of total body weight)
  2. In patients with circulatory overload:
     a. Increased plasma volume increases mean arterial pressure. The myocardium stretches to accommodate the larger blood volume, the cardiac output is correspondingly increased, and plasma hydrostatic pressure also increases beyond normal values.
     b. If cardiac status is compromised or if the isotonic hypervolemia continues for a prolonged period, the heart cannot handle the excess volume. This results in congestive heart failure (CHF) and edema.
     c. When a patient's intravascular space becomes overloaded

with fluid, eventually the heart will not be able to accommodate the blood.

    d. As a result of CHF, the FVE progresses into the pulmonary edema, which is life-threatening.

    e. Symptoms include elevated blood pressure, bounding pulse, and neck vein distention.

  2. In patients with interstitial edema:

    a. A higher plasma hydrostatic pressure forces a higher-than-normal outflow of fluid from the capillaries into the tissue spaces.

    b. Fluid can accumulate subcutaneously in dependent parts of the body; this is peripheral edema.

    c. Fluid accumulating in the lungs is heard as moist crackles on auscultation.

D. Potential nursing diagnoses

  1. Fluid Volume Excess

  2. High Risk for Ineffective Breathing Pattern

  3. Decreased Cardiac Output

E. Interventions

  1. Medical management involves:

    a. Prescription of diuretics to enhance water excretion by the kidneys

    b. Restriction of oral fluid and salt intake

    c. Titration of IV fluid volume composition and intake

    d. Treatment of contributory underlying disease states (eg, in CHF, digoxin would be prescribed to increase cardiac output)

  2. Nursing considerations:

    a. Assess cardiovascular status (eg, pulse rate and quality, blood pressure, neck vein filling).

    b. Monitor hemodynamic parameters, such as cardiac output and intracardiac pressures.

    c. Assess respiratory status; auscultate breath sounds, and monitor rate and ease of breathing.

    d. Monitor for weight gain in relation to total body weight; estimate a gain of 1 L of fluid for every kilogram (2.2 lb) of increased weight.

    e. Measure and record daily weights.

    f. Monitor for the presence of peripheral edema. Check for pitting edema by pressing gently with a fingertip into edematous area; if depression remains, the depth of the "pit" indicates severity of the edema.

    g. Monitor laboratory values; decreased hematocrit and BUN may indicate isotonic FVE.

    h. Monitor intake and output.

       i.   Position the patient comfortably to relieve respiratory symptoms, edema, and pressure.

       j.   Evaluate the patient's knowledge of the prescribed diet or medication regimen; assess for any dietary factors that may have led to FVE.

       k.   Refer the patient to a dietitian for nutritional consultation.

F. **Evaluation**

   1.   The patient's breath sounds, breathing patterns, vital signs, and urinary output are normal.

   2.   The patient displays no signs of edema.

   3.   The patient's fluid volume status is normal.

   4.   The patient's cardiac output is normal.

VI. Hypotonic FVE

A. **Description**

   1.   Hypotonic FVE, sometimes called *water intoxication*, is an increase in water volume without a corresponding increase in sodium concentration, producing hypo-osmolar ECF.

   2.   Fluid shifts into the cells from the ECF, causing water logging of cells.

B. **Etiology**

   1.   Hypotonic FVE results from:

       a.   Excess oral intake of water or IV fluid therapy with hypotonic solutions (eg, 5% dextrose and water)

       b.   Underlying medical conditions that impair normal fluid excretion, including cardiac disease (in which there is insufficient arterial pressure for normal renal perfusion); syndrome of inappropriate ADH (SIADH) secretion resulting from extreme stress, benign and cancerous central nervous system (CNS) lesions, or fever; overuse of drugs, such as corticosteroids

       c.   Loss of isotonic fluids (through vomiting, burns, hemorrhage) combined with replacement of water but not sodium and other lost solutes

   2.   Hypotonic FVE always involves an osmotic fluid shift from the ECF into the ICF (cell swelling).

C. **Assessment findings**

   1.   Weight gain

   2.   Thirst

   3.   Excretion of dilute urine

   4.   Nonpitting edema

   5.   Dysrythmias secondary to decreased plasma sodium and potassium

   6.   Low sodium levels

   7.   Symptoms of cerebral ICF excess, including:

       a.   Nausea

       b. Malaise

       c. Lethargy

       d. Headache

       e. Seizures, coma, and death if ICF fluid shift into brain cells is not reversed

D. Potential nursing diagnoses

    1. Fluid Volume Excess

    2. High Risk for Decreased Cardiac Output

    3. High Risk for Injury

E. Interventions

    1. Medical management involves:

       a. Restriction of water intake to a volume that is less than urine output

       b. Increasing salt in the diet

       c. Administration of IV hypertonic (3%) saline solutions for severe hyponatremia (eg, sodium concentration of 110 mEq/L or less). Note that hypertonic solutions are only given if the patient's life is threatened and should be used cautiously to avoid overcorrection of the sodium loss; plasma sodium should not rise above 145 to 150 mEq/L.

    2. Nursing considerations are the same as for isotonic FVE (see Section V.D.2), plus the following:

       a. Monitor for abnormal water-seeking behavior such as may be seen in patients with psychological disorders (psychogenic polydipsia) or in those whose thirst regulation has been altered by disease process (primary polydipsia).

       b. Assess neurologic status for signs of ICF excess.

F. Evaluation

    1. The patient's urinary output and cardiac output are normal.

    2. The patient's level of consciousness is normal.

    3. The patient is free from injury.

VII. Hypertonic FVE

A. Description

    1. Hypertonic FVE is an increase in sodium concentration with water volume remaining normal.

    2. This results in ECF that is hyperosmolar compared with normal plasma and tissue fluids.

    3. ICF shifts into the ECF.

B. Etiology

    1. Hypertonic FVE results from:

       a. Excess intake of hypertonic fluids, such as salty liquids or seawater

       b. Excess solute (eg, sodium) retention secondary to impaired regulatory mechanisms or disease process.

    2. It always involves an osmotic fluid shift from the ICF to the ECF (cell shrinkage).

C. **Assessment findings**
    1. Clinical manifestations relate to the effect of the excess solute in the ECF combined with FVE; symptoms of hypertonic FVE are the same as for isotonic FVE (see Section V.C).
    2. ICF deficit is manifested by neurologic symptoms (eg, decreased level of consciousness [LOC], lethargy, muscle twitching, possible seizures, and coma); symptom severity is related to the speed with which plasma sodium concentration rises, with its subsequent osmotic dehydration of cerebral cells.
    3. Hypernatremia is present.

D. **Potential nursing diagnoses**
    1. Fluid Volume Excess
    2. High Risk for Injury
    3. High Risk for Decreased Cardiac Output

E. **Interventions**
    1. Medical management involves:
        a. Treatment of underlying disease (eg, renal failure or CNS lesion)
        b. Discontinuing or removing the source of the hypertonic fluid intake
        c. Removal of excess sodium by diuretics
        d. Correction of the ICF water deficit (plus water lost with diuretic therapy) through replacement with oral water or hypotonic IV solution
        e. Treatment of the symptoms of the high ECF solute and the ICF deficit
    2. Nursing considerations are the same as for isotonic FVE (see Section V.D.2), plus the following:
        a. Assess LOC, neuromuscular status, presence or absence of tremors, and rigidity to detect any signs of ICF deficit.
        b. Provide patient teaching regarding prevention through dietary modifications, avoidance of high-salt foods, and self-monitoring of symptoms (eg, rapid weight gain, presence of edema).

F. **Evaluation**
    1. The patient's LOC is normal.
    2. The patient's urinary output, vital signs, and breath sounds are normal.
    3. The patient's fluid volume status is normal.
    4. The patient's cardiac output is normal.
    5. The patient is free from injury (Table 3–1).

TABLE 3–1.
Changes in extracellular fluid volume and plasma sodium concentration as determinants of body fluid balance

TYPE OF ECF FLUID VOLUME IMBALANCE	ECF VOLUME	ECF SOLUTE CONCENTRATION Na^+ (mEq)	ICF VOLUME (CELLS SWELL OR SHRINK)	ICF SOLUTE CONCENTRATION K^+ (mEq)
Isotonic FVE H_2O gain = Na^+ gain	↑	No change	No change	No change
Hypertonic FVE Na^+ gain > H_2O gain	↑	↑	Cells shrink	↑
Hypertonic FVE H_2O gain > Na^+ gain	↑	↓	Cells swell	↓
Isotonic FVD H_2O loss = Na^+ loss	↓	No change	No change	No change
Hypertonic FVD H_2O loss > Na^+ loss	↓	↑	Cells shrink	↑
Hypotonic FVD Na^+ loss > H_2O loss	↓	↓	Cells swell	↓

Key: ECF, extracellular fluid; ICF, intracellular fluid; FVE, fluid volume excess; FVD, fluid volume deficit.

Bibliography

Brunner, L., & Suddarth, D. (1988). *Textbook of medical-surgical nursing* (6th ed.). Philadelphia: J.B. Lippincott.

Guyton, A. (1991). *Textbook of medical physiology* (8th ed.). Philadelphia: W.B. Saunders.

Ignatavicius, D., & Bayne, M. (1991). *Medical-surgical nursing: A nursing process approach.* Philadelphia: W.B. Saunders.

Kinney, M., Packa, D., & Dunbar, S. (1993). *AACN's clinical reference for critical-care nursing* (3rd ed.). St. Louis: C.V. Mosby.

Kokko, J., & Tannen, R. (1990). *Fluid and electrolytes* (2nd ed.). Philadelphia: W.B. Saunders.

Metheny, N. (1992). *Fluid and electrolyte balance: Nursing considerations* (2nd ed.). Philadelphia: J.B. Lippincott.

Rose, D. (1989). *Clinical physiology of acid-base and electrolyte disorders* (3rd ed.). New York: McGraw-Hill.

STUDY QUESTIONS

1. In which of the following types of fluid volume deficit (FVD) does water volume remain normal?
   a. isotonic FVD
   b. hypotonic FVD
   c. hypertonic FVD
   d. allatonic FVD

2. When monitoring a patient with a isotonic FVD, the nurse is aware that the minimum urine output is:
   a. 10 mL/hour
   b. 20 mL/hour
   c. 30 mL/hour
   d. 40 mL/hour

3. The phenomenon of third-space fluid shifting involves:
   a. iso-osmolar fluid shifts into body cavities where the fluid is not available for exchange with plasma volume
   b. the three types of fluid volume deficits
   c. hypoosmolar fluid shifts into the extracellular fluid
   d. iatrogenic fluid shifts into the lymphatic system

4. In patients with isotonic fluid volume excess (FVE) and circulating overload, the potential outcome is:
   a. cell swelling
   b. cerebral cell dehydration
   c. water intoxication
   d. congestive heart failure (CHF)

5. The physician has ordered administration of a hypertonic saline solution. The nurse would administer:
   a. 3% saline solution
   b. 0.33% saline solution
   c. 0.45% saline solution
   d. 0.9% saline solution

6. Third-space fluid accumulation may occur in the:
   a. peritoneal cavity
   b. pleural space
   c. interstitial space
   d. all of the above

7. Which of the following is a potential nursing diagnosis for a patient with isotonic FVD?
   a. Increased cardiac output
   b. Decreased cardiac output
   c. Fluid volume excess
   d. Altered urinary habits

8. When assessing a patient with hypotonic FVE, the nurse can expect to find:
   a. hyponatremia
   b. confusion
   c. headache
   d. all of the above

ANSWER KEY

1. **Correct response: b**
   Hypotonic FVD involves a decrease in solute concentration with water volume remaining normal.
   a. Isotonic FVD involves an equal decrease in ECF solute concentration and water volume.
   c. Hypertonic FVD involves a decrease in water volume without a corresponding decrease in solute concentration.
   d. There is no such entity.
   Analysis/Physiologic/Assessment

2. **Correct response: c**
   Urine output should be a bare minimum of 30 mL/hour or 500 to 700 ml/day.
   a, b, and d. These responses are incorrect.
   Comprehension/Safe Care/Evaluation

3. **Correct response: a**
   Third-space fluid shifting involves iso-osmolar fluid shifts into spaces other than the ICF or ECF where the fluid is not available for exchanges with plasma.
   b, c, and d. These responses are incorrect.
   Analysis/Physiologic/Analysis

4. **Correct response: d**
   In patients with circulatory overload due to isotonic FVE, the excess volume cannot be managed and results in CHF and edema.
   a. Cell shrinking, not swelling, occurs.
   b and c. These responses are incorrect.
   Application/Safe Care/Evaluation

5. **Correct response: a**
   Hypertonic fluid has a greater concentration of sodium to water volume. A 3% saline solution has a higher concentration than a 0.33%, 0.45%, or 0.9% saline solution.
   b, c, and d. These responses are incorrect.
   Application/Safe Care/Implementation

6. **Correct response: d**
   Third-space fluid accumulation refers to the accumulation of fluid in spaces that are not part of the circulation. These spaces include the peritoneal cavity, pleural space, and interstitial space.
   Comprehension/Physiologic/Assessment

7. **Correct response: b**
   Isotonic FVD may change cardiac output because as fluid is lost, cardiac output tends to drop. Assessment findings characteristic of FVD could also include decreased blood pressure and tachycardia.
   a. This response is incorrect.
   c. Fluid volume excess is the direct opposite of fluid volume deficit.
   d. Altered urinary habits is not a potential nursing diagnosis.
   Application/Safe Care/Analysis

8. **Correct response: d**
   Symptoms of hypotonic FVE are hyponatremia, confusion, and headache. Other symptoms include nausea, malaise, lethargy, weight gain, thirst, and non-pitting edema.
   Analysis/Safe Care/Assessment

Electrolyte Balance

I. Overview of electrolytes

A. Description

1. Electrolytes are solutes that are found in body fluids (eg, intracellular fluid [ICF] and extracellular fluid [ECF]).

2. When dissolved in solution, electrolytes form *ions*:
   a. Positively charged ions are called *cations*.
   b. Negatively charged ions are called *anions*.

3. Major body electrolytes include:
   a. Sodium (Na^+)–cation
   b. Potassium (K^+)–cation
   c. Chloride (Cl^-)–anion
   d. Calcium (Ca^+)–cation
   e. Magnesium (Mg^+)–cation
   f. Phosphorus (P^-)–anion
   g. Hydrogen (H^+)–cation
   h. Bicarbonate (HCO_3^-)–anion

B. Sources of electrolytes

1. Normal sources of electrolyte intake include all foods and fluids.

2. Abnormal sources of electrolyte intake include:
   a. Medications
   b. Intravenous solutions
   c. Hyperalimentation

C. Role of electrolytes

1. Electrolytes conduct electricity across cell membranes; they are needed for life processes to occur.

    2. Electrolytes function to:
        a. Maintain osmolality of body fluid compartments
        b. Regulate balance of acids and bases
        c. Aid in neurologic and neuromuscular conduction

  D. **Balance of electrolytes**
    1. For a homeostatic condition to exist, equal amounts of anions and cations must be present on either side of the cell membrane (Fig. 4–1); this is known as electrical neutrality.
    2. Electrolytes will move from one side of the cell membrane to another in an attempt to maintain an electrically neutral state.
    3. Extracellular electrolytes are found in the interstitial and intravascular fluids where there is a balance of cations and anions.

II. Electrolyte distribution and excretion
  A. **Distribution**
    1. Electrolyte distribution varies between the ICF and ECF
    2. ICF electrolytes include:
        a. Potassium, the chief cation
        b. Phosphorus, the chief anion
        c. Large amount of protein
        d. Small amounts of magnesium, calcium, sulfate, and bicarbonate (Table 4–1).
        e. Extremely small amounts of sodium and chloride
    3. ECF electrolytes include:
        a. Sodium, the chief cation
        b. Chloride, the chief anion

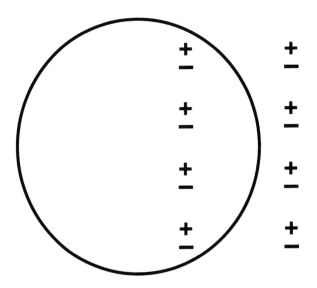

FIGURE 4–1.
Electrical neutrality.

TABLE 4–1.
Approximation of Major Electrolyte Content
in Intracellular Fluid

ELECTROLYTES	mEq/L
Cations:	
Potassium (K+)	150
Magnesium (Mg^{2+})	40
Sodium (Na$^+$)	10
Total cations	200
Anions:	
Phosphates }	150
Sulfates	
Bicarbonate (HCO$_3^-$)	10
Proteinate	40
Total anions	200

Metheny, N. M. (1992). Fluid and Electrolyte Balance (2nd ed.). J.B. Lippincott.

    c. Bicarbonate
    d. Small amounts of potassium, calcium, magnesium, sulfate, and phosphorus
    e. Protein in an amount smaller than in the ECF (Table 4–2).
  5. The concentration of electrolytes in body fluids can be expressed as *milliequivalents per liter (mEq/L)* or *milligrams per deciliter (mg/dL)*.
  6. The ECF includes intravascular and interstitial fluids; the interstitial fluid has essentially the same electrolyte distribution as the intravascular fluid, but it is not measurable.
  7. ICF electrolytes are found in the intracellular space only and are not measurable; their values can be inferred only from ECF values.
  8. The concentration of specific electrolytes can be measured using serum or urine tests (Table 4–3).
B. **Excretion**
  1. Electrolytes are lost during excessive elimination of body fluids for any reason.
  2. Renal excretion of electrolytes is abnormal when diuretics are used.
  3. Gastrointestinal (GI) elimination of electrolytes is abnormal when diarrhea is present.
  4. In upper GI tract fluid elimination, hydrogen and potassium tend to be lost.

TABLE 4–2.
Plasma Electrolytes

ELECTROLYTES	mEq/L
Cations:	
Sodium (Na$^+$)	142
Potassium (K$^+$)	5
Calcium (Ca^{2+})	5
Magnesium (Mg^{2+})	2
Total cations	154
Anions:	
Chloride (Cl$^-$)	103
Bicarbonate (HCO$_3^-$)	26
Phosphate (HPO$_4^{2-}$)	2
Sulfate (SO$_4^{2-}$)	1
Organic acids	5
Proteinate	17
Total anions	154

Metheny, N. M. (1992). Fluid and Electrolyte Balance (2nd ed.). J.B. Lippincott.

5. In lower GI tract fluid elimination, bicarbonate tends to be lost.
6. Excessive diaphoresis contributes to sodium and chloride loss.
7. Surgical drains also may contribute to excessive electrolyte loss.

III. Electrolyte regulation
A. Renal regulation
1. Electrolytes are regulated mainly by the kidneys and the endocrine system.
2. In the kidneys, electrolytes are balanced by glomerular filtration, tubular reabsorption and secretion.
   a. The process of glomerular filtration can be compared to filtration that occurs outside of the body (i.e., filtration of coffee).
   b. Water goes through the filter and takes smaller substances along with it, leaving the larger substances behind in the filter (i.e., in the example of coffee filter, water will take the color and flavor of the coffee, leaving the larger grounds behind in the filter.)
   c. The glomerulus provides the same functions.
   d. It is a filter that leaves the larger molecules (protein, red and white blood cells) in the blood stream while filtering out the smaller molecules (electrolytes, waste products).

TABLE 4–3.
Laboratory Tests Used to Evaluate Fluid and Electrolyte Status

TEST	USUAL REFERENCE RANGE
Serum sodium	136–145 mEq/L
Serum potassium	3.5–5.0 mEq/L
Total serum calcium	8.5–10.5 mg/dl (approximately 50% in ionized form)
Serum magnesium	1.3–2.1 mEq/L
Serum phosphorus	2.5–4.5 mg/dL
Serum chloride	95–108 mEq/L
Carbon dioxide content	24–30 mEq/L
Serum osmolality	280–295 mOsm/kg
Blood urea nitrogen (BUN)	10–20 mg/dL
Serum creatinine	0.7–1.5 mg/dL
BUN: Creatinine ratio	10:1
Hematocrit	Male: 44% –52%
	Female: 39%–47%
Serum glucose	70–110 mg/dL
Serum albumin	3.5–5.5 g/dL
Urinary sodium	80–180 mEq/day
Urinary potassium	40–80 mEq/day
Urinary chloride	110–250 mEq/day
Urinary specific gravity	1.003–1.035
Urine osmolality	
Extreme range:	50–1400 mOsm/L
Typical urine:	500–800 mOsm/L
Urinary pH	4.5–8.0
Typical urine:	<6.6

Smeltzer and Bare. Brunner and Suddarth's Textbook of Medical-Surgical Nursing *(7th ed.). (1992), J.B. Lippincott.*

3. Blood is filtered through the glomerulus, and water and electrolytes enter the renal tubules.
4. The majority of electrolytes are reabsorbed in the proximal tubule,
   but reabsorption occurs along the entire length of the tubule.
   a. Tubular reabsorption can be compared with a sponge.
   b. Water is reabsorbed through specialized cells that line the
      tubules.
   c. The amount of water reabsorbed depends on the amount
      needed by the body.
   d. As water moves through the length of the tubule, there is
      less water present for reabsorption at the distal ends than in
      the proximal ends.
   e. In the distal and collecting tubules, water is reabsorbed only

in the presence of anti-diuretic hormone (which is released when the body needs more water).

   f. As water is reabsorbed through the length of the tubules, electrolytes are also reabsorbed.

   g. Electrolytes move from one side of the tubular membrane to the other in order to maintain electrical neutrality. (Fig. 4–2).

   5. *Electrolyte secretion* occurs when an electrolyte moves from the blood into the tubule, as opposed to entering the tubule through glomerular filtration.

   6. Some electrolytes are regulated by secretion and reabsorption.

C. **Endocrine regulation**

   1. Along with the kidneys, the endocrine system is the primary regulator of electrolytes.

   2. Pituitary adrenocorticotropic hormone stimulation enhances adrenal release of aldosterone.

   3. Aldosterone acts on the tubules to reabsorb sodium.

   4. When sodium is reabsorbed, another positively charged electrolyte—the cation potassium—is secreted into the tubules for excretion.

D. **Gastrointestinal regulation**

   1. Electrolytes are secreted, absorbed, and exchanged in the GI tract.

   2. Gastric juices are high in acid content, and the exchange between anions and cations occurs across the small bowel (Tables 4–1 and 4–2 and Figs. 4–1 and 4–2).

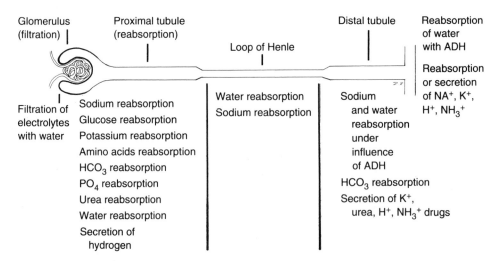

FIGURE 4–2.
Reabsorption and secretion of electrolytes along the kidney tubule.

Bibliography

Alspach, J. G. (1991). *Core curriculum for critical care nursing* (4th ed.). Philadelphia: W.B. Saunders.

Brunner, L. S., & Suddarth, D. S. (1992). *Textbook of medical-surgical nursing* (7th ed.). Philadelphia: J.B. Lippincott.

Guyton, A. (1991). *Textbook of medical physiology* (8th ed.). Philadelphia: W.B. Saunders.

McCance, K. L., & Huether, S. E. (1994). *Pathophysiology: The biologic basis for disease in adults and children* (2nd ed.). St. Louis: Mosby–Year Book.

Metheny, N. (1992). *Fluid and electrolyte balance: Nursing considerations* (2nd ed.). Philadelphia: J.B. Lippincott.

STUDY QUESTIONS

1. Electrolytes are responsible for all of the following functions *except:*
   a. maintaining the osmolality of body fluid compartments
   b. regulating the balance of acids and bases
   c. aiding in neurologic and neuromuscular conduction
   d. regulating body fluids

2. Major intracellular fluid (ICF) electrolytes include:
   a. sodium
   b. potassium
   c. chloride
   d. bicarbonate

3. Primary ACTH stimulation will result in:
   a. sodium reabsorption
   b. sodium excretion
   c. potassium reabsorption
   d. decreased aldosterone release

4. When caring for a patient who has had a small bowel resection and is 1-day postoperative, the nurse is aware that the patient is at risk for electrolyte imbalance because of:
   a. impaired nutrient intake
   b. impaired exchange between anions and cations

   c. pain
   d. impaired endocrine stimulation

5. Cations are defined as:
   a. positively charged ions
   b. negatively charged ions
   c. enzyme-like substances
   d. precursors of electrolytes

6. The chief cation found in the extracellular fluid (ECF) is:
   a. sodium
   b. potassium
   c. chloride
   d. phosphorus

7. Which of the following statements is *not* true?
   a. ICF electrolytes are found within the cell membrane.
   b. ICF electrolytes are not measurable.
   c. ICF electrolytes have a non-variable concentration.
   d. ICF electrolyte values are inferred from ECF values.

8. Which of the following sources is a normal source of electrolyte intake?
   a. medications
   b. Gatorade
   c. IV solutions
   d. hyperalimentation

ANSWER KEY

1. *Correct response: d*
   Electrolytes do not play a primary role in the regulation of body fluids.
   a, b, and c. Electrolytes do maintain body fluid osmolality, regulate the balance of acid and bases, and aid in neurologic conduction.
   Knowledge/Physiologic/NA

2. *Correct response: b*
   Potassium is the major cation found in the ICF.
   a, c, and d. Sodium, chloride, and bicarbonate are found in greater amounts in the ECF.
   Knowledge/Physiologic/Assessment

3. *Correct response: a*
   Stimulation of ACTH will result in increased aldosterone release and, therefore, increased sodium reabsorption.
   b. Sodium is reabsorbed, not excreted.
   c. Potassium will be excreted as sodium is reabsorbed.
   d. Aldosterone release is increased with ACTH.
   Knowledge/Physiologic/Analysis

4. *Correct response: b*
   Gastrointestinal balance of electrolytes involves the exchange of cations and anions in the small bowel; surgery would interfere with this for a period of time.
   a. Nutrient intake refers to the ability to eat.
   c. Pain does not alter electrolyte balance.

   d. There is no endocrine impairment associated with bowel surgery.
   Application/Physiologic/Analysis

5. *Correct response: a*
   Cations are positively charged ions.
   b. Anions are negatively charged ions.
   c and d. These responses are incorrect.
   Knowledge/Physiologic/NA

6. *Correct response: a*
   Sodium is the primary cation found in the ECF.
   b. Potassium is the chief cation of the ICF.
   c and d. These are anions.
   Knowledge/Physiologic/Assessment

7. *Correct response: c*
   ICF electrolyte concentrations fluctuate based on normal and abnormal occurrences. Electrolytes will move from one side of a cell membrane to another to maintain neutrality.
   a, b and d. These are true statements.
   Knowledge/Physiologic/NA

8. *Correct response: b*
   Food and fluids are normal sources of electrolytes for humans.
   a, c, and d. These are abnormal sources necessary for patients who experience electrolyte deficits.
   Knowledge/Health Promotion/Planning

Sodium: Normal and Altered Balance

I.   Normal balance

A.   Description

1.   Sodium is the major extracellular fluid (ECF) cation.
2.   Normal serum sodium concentration ranges from 136 to 145 mEq/L.
3.   Sodium is regulated proportionally with water and chloride.

B.   Supply and sources

1.   Most sodium is found outside of the cell in the ECF where it can be measured by serum tests.
2.   Some sodium is found in the intracellular fluid (ICF), but it is not measurable.
3.   Sodium is taken in through the diet. The minimum sodium requirement for adults is 2 g daily; most adults consume more because sodium is abundant in almost all foods.

C.   Functions

1.   Because sodium is found in abundance in the ECF, its balance is important for many physiologic functions, including:

a. Facilitating impulse transmission in nerve and muscle fibers by participating in the sodium-potassium pump

b. Influencing the levels of potassium and chloride by exchanging for potassium and attracting to chloride

c. Assisting in acid–base balance by combining with bicarbonate and chloride

2. Sodium also determines the volume and osmolality of the ECF and regulates body water.

D. Regulation

1. Sodium is lost through the skin, gastrointestinal tract, and genitourinary tract.

2. Renal and endocrine mechanisms contribute to sodium balance.

3. The kidneys match sodium excretion to sodium intake:

a. Through glomerular filtration, sodium passes through the glomerular filter along with water.

b. Through tubular reabsorption, sodium is reabsorbed with water along the course of the tubules, mostly in the proximal tubule. The presence of aldosterone in the tubules will enhance reabsorption of sodium.

4. The endocrine system secretes aldosterone and antidiuretic hormone (ADH) to help regulate sodium levels and maintain the balance between sodium and water:

a. When ECF sodium is decreased, the adrenal glands send aldosterone to the kidneys, where sodium is reabsorbed.

b. When ECF sodium is increased, aldosterone secretion is decreased, allowing sodium excretion.

c. When ECF sodium is elevated, ECF osmolality also is elevated, and ADH is secreted; this increases tubular reabsorption of water.

d. Decreased ECF sodium reduces ECF osmolality.

e. Pituitary secretion of adrenocorticotropin hormone helps regulate sodium by increasing the presence of aldosterone.

II. Sodium deficiency: Hyponatremia

A. Description: Serum sodium levels below 136 mEq/L

B. Etiology

1. Sodium loss in excess of water, such as from:

a. Prolonged diuretic therapy (which impairs sodium reabsorption in Henle's loop)

b. Excessive burns (which cause a large loss of ECF, where sodium concentration is high)

c. Excessive diaphoresis (because sodium is found in large amounts in sweat)

d. Prolonged vomiting, nasogastric suction, diarrhea, or laxative abuse

e. Renal disease

2. Water gain in excess of sodium, such as from:
   a. Excessive administration of water, as in intravenous solutions, such as D_5W; eventually water will shift into the ICF in an attempt to balance the ratio of sodium to water (Fig. 5–1).
   b. Compulsive water drinking that occurs with some psychiatric disorders; this results in diluted sodium levels and allows water to shift into the cells.
3. Inadequate intake or absorption, such as due to anorexia or acute alcoholism
4. Adrenal insufficiency, in which aldosterone levels are low and sodium reabsorption becomes compromised, thus allowing sodium excretion
5. Syndrome of inappropriate ADH (SIADH), in which water is retained and dilutional hyponatremia occurs

C. **Assessment findings**
   1. Clinical manifestations may include vomiting and diarrhea; however, these symptoms may actually be the cause of hyponatremia.
   2. Neurologic and musculoskeletal symptoms may occur because sodium is required for normal functioning of these systems; such symptoms may include:
      a. Muscle cramps
      b. Muscle twitching
      c. Headache
      d. Dizziness
      e. Confusion
      f. Convulsions
      g. Coma
   3. Because sodium is required for regulation of ECF volume and balance of ECF water, water shifts from the ECF to the ICF, causing cells to swell and resulting in central nervous system (CNS) symptoms.
   4. As sodium is lost, the serum becomes more concentrated. Laboratory tests reveal:
      a. Serum sodium level below 136 mEq/L
      b. Urine specific gravity > 1.010
      c. Serum osmolality > 285 mOsm/kg.

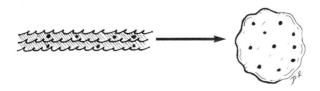

FIGURE 5–1.
Hyponatremia. When water is present in excess of sodium, water will move into the cell, causing it to swell.

D. **Potential nursing diagnoses**
1. Fluid Volume Excess related to excessive body water
2. High Risk for Injury related to confusion

E. **Interventions**
1. Prevent hyponatremia or ensure early detection by identifying high-risk patients (eg, those receiving diuretic therapy or undergoing gastric suctioning and those with renal disorders, burn injuries, or fever) and providing appropriate patient education.
2. Aid in the treatment objective of restoring serum sodium level.
3. Restrict water intake to allow sodium and water to balance naturally.
4. Administer hypertonic solutions (eg, 3% normal saline) *with caution*; these solutions will force water to leave the ICF to balance the sodium instilled in the ECF, thus causing cellular shrinkage.
5. Measure and record daily weights to track fluid retention and loss.
6. Monitor vital signs and serum sodium levels.

F. **Evaluation**
1. Serum sodium level returns to a range between 136 and 145 mEq/L.
2. The patient remains free of symptoms.

III. **Sodium excess: Hypernatremia**

A. **Description: Serum sodium level above 145 mEq/L**

B. **Etiology**
1. Sodium gain in excess of water, such as from:
   a. Administration of hypertonic parenteral solutions or tube feedings
   b. Excessive dietary intake of sodium, which may occur through the normal route or through parenteral and enteral feedings
2. Water loss in excess of sodium, such as from:
   a. Severe watery stool
   b. Severe insensible water loss
   c. Burns
   d. Osmotic diuresis
   e. Diabetes insipidus
3. Fluid shifts:
   a. In certain conditions, water will shift out of the ICF into the ECF to balance the excess ECF sodium.
   b. This causes the cells to shrink as they lose water volume (Fig. 5–2).

C. **Assessment findings**
1. Symptoms of hypernatremia often are associated with those of dehydration, including:

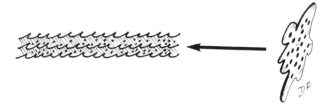

FIGURE 5–2.
Hypernatremia. When sodium is present in excess of water, water will move out of the cell, causing the cell to shrink.

    a. Thirst
    b. Tachycardia
    c. Dry mucous membranes
    d. Lethargy

  2. Because sodium is required for normal neurologic and musculoskeletal conduction, hypernatremia commonly has CNS manifestations, including:
    a. Hyperactive reflexes
    b. Lethargy
    c. Seizures

  3. As sodium is retained or fluid shifts, the serum becomes more dilute; laboratory tests reveal:
    a. Serum sodium level > 145 mEq/L
    b. Urine specific gravity > 1.015
    c. Serum osmolality > 295 mOsm/kg

D. Potential nursing diagnoses
  1. Fluid Volume Deficit related to sodium–water imbalances
  2. High Risk for Injury related to lethargy

E. Interventions
  1. Identify high-risk patients (eg, those receiving hypertonic tube feedings or hypertonic total parenteral nutrition [TPN] solutions), and provide appropriate patient education.
  2. Aid in the treatment objective of reducing the serum sodium level.
  3. Measure and record daily weights to monitor fluid retention and loss.
  4. Record intake and output because the patient may have a markedly decreased output.
  5. Assess vital signs.
  6. Assess mentation.
  7. Administer parenteral solutions *with caution*; hypotonic sodium solutions (*except* D_5W) are best to prevent fluid overload.

   8. Monitor laboratory tests.
   9. Ensure adequate water intake if a patient is receiving hypertonic fluid to prevent solute overload (eg, dilute tube feedings and be sure to infuse TPN at prescribed rate).
 F. Evaluation
   1. Serum sodium level returns to a range between 136 and 145 mEq/L.
   2. The patient remains free of symptoms.

Bibliography

Brunner, L., & Suddarth, D. (1988). *Textbook of medical-surgical nursing* (6th ed.). Philadelphia: J.B. Lippincott.

Guyton, A. (1991). *Textbook of medical physiology* (8th ed.). Philadelphia: W.B. Saunders.

Ignatavicius, D., & Bayne, M. (1991). *Medical-surgical nursing: A nursing process approach.* Philadelphia: W.B. Saunders.

Kinney, M., Packa, D., & Dunbar, S. (1993). *AACN's clinical reference for critical-care nursing* (3rd ed.). St. Louis: C.V. Mosby.

Kokko, J., & Tannen, R. (1990). *Fluid and electrolytes* (2nd ed.). Philadelphia: W.B. Saunders.

Metheny, N. (1992). *Fluid and electrolyte balance: Nursing considerations* (2nd ed.). Philadelphia: J.B. Lippincott.

Rose, D. (1989). *Clinical physiology of acid-base and electrolyte disorders* (3rd ed.). New York: McGraw-Hill.

STUDY QUESTIONS

1. When assessing a patient for hypernatremia, the nurse would expect to find:
   a. serum sodium level of 135 mEq/liter
   b. moist mucous membranes
   c. thirst
   d. hypoactive reflexes

2. Which of the following IV solutions would the nurse administer for a patient with hypernatremia?
   a. 3% saline
   b. 0.33% saline
   c. D_5W
   d. lactated Ringer's solution

3. When ECF sodium is decreased, the adrenal glands send aldosterone to the kidneys to:
   a. increase sodium reabsorption
   b. decrease sodium reabsorption
   c. increase water reabsorption
   d. decrease water reabsorption

4. Patients at high risk for hyponatremia include all of the following *except:*
   a. patients receiving hypertonic TPN
   b. patients on diuretic therapy
   c. burn victims
   d. patients with gastric suctioning

5. The nurse should administer hypertonic IV solutions with caution because these solutions will force:
   a. water to leave the ECF
   b. water to leave the ICF
   c. cellular swelling
   d. hydrostatic pressure to drop

6. Aldosterone reabsorption of sodium occurs after stimulation with:
   a. Adrenocorticotropic hormone (ACTH)
   b. insulin
   c. antidiuretic hormone (ADH)
   d. pitocin

7. When caring for a patient with hyponatremia, the nurse is careful to restrict:
   a. water
   b. sodium
   c. potassium
   d. chloride

8. When caring for a patient with hypernatremia, the nurse is careful to administer:
   a. water
   b. sodium
   c. potassium
   d. chloride

ANSWER KEY

1. **Correct response: c**
   Thirst and other signs of dehydration indicate hypernatremia.
   a. Serum sodium level is greater than 145 mEq/liter in hypernatremia.
   b. Dry, not moist mucous membranes are found in hypernatremia.
   c. Reflexes are hyperactive, not hypoactive in hypernatremia.
   Knowledge/Safe Care/Assessment

2. **Correct response: b**
   Hypotonic solutions are prescribed for a patient with hypernatremia; 0.33% saline is hypotonic.
   b. 3% saline solution is hypertonic.
   c. D_5W is contraindicated because of the possibility of fluid overload.
   d. This response is incorrect.
   Knowledge/Safe Care/Implementation

3. **Correct response: a**
   When ECF sodium is decreased, the adrenal glands send aldosterone to the kidneys to increase sodium reabsorption in an attempt to balance sodium levels.
   b, c, and d. These responses are incorrect.
   Analysis/Physiologic/Analysis

4. **Correct response: a**
   Patients receiving hypertonic TPN are at risk to develop hypernatremia.
   b, c, and d. Patients on diuretic therapy, burn victims, and patients having gastric suctioning are all at increased risk for developing hyponatremia.
   Comprehension/Safe Care/Assessment

5. **Correct response: b**
   Hypertonic IV fluids will force water to leave the ICF to balance the sodium in the ECF, thus causing cell shrinkage.
   a, c and d. These responses are incorrect.
   Application/Safe Care/Implementation

6. **Correct response: a**
   Adrenocorticotropic hormone (ACTH) is released from the pituitary; it stimulates adrenal release of aldosterone.
   b, c, and d. These do not influence sodium reabsorption.
   Knowledge/Physiologic/Analysis

7. **Correct response: a**
   In hyponatremia, water is present in excessive amounts.
   b, c, and d. These are electrolyte replacements and are not suitable treatment choices for hyponatremia.
   Application/Safe Care/Implementation

8. **Correct response: a**
   Patients with hypernatremia are thirsty; they need water replacement to balance the rising sodium levels.
   b, c, and d. These are not appropriate treatments for hypernatremia.
   Application/Safe Care/Analysis

Potassium: Normal and Altered Balance

I. Normal balance

A. Description

1. Potassium is the major cation in intracellular fluid (ICF).
2. Normal serum potassium concentration ranges from 3.5 to 5.0 mEq/L.

B. Supply and sources

1. Potassium is taken in through the diet; it is found abundantly in citrus fruits, vegetables, chocolate, and licorice.
2. Abnormal routes of potassium intake include intravenous (IV) solutions and nutritional supplements.
3. Potassium is lost from the gastrointestinal (GI) and renal systems.
4. Abnormal amounts of potassium are lost through the excess elimination of urine and stool.
5. Ninety-eight percent of all potassium is found inside the cell; 2% is found in extracellular fluid (ECF). This 2% is reflected in serum concentration measurements.

Paradiso, C: *Lippincott's Review Series: Fluids and Electrolytes* © 1995 J. B. Lippincott Company

C. Functions

1. Because potassium is positively charged and is found in the ICF, its balance is important for several physiologic functions, including:

   a. Regulating osmolarity of ECF by exchanging with sodium
   b. Maintaining the transmembrane electrical potential that exists between the ICF and ECF
   c. Maintaining normal neuromuscular contraction by participation in the sodium-potassium pump
   d. Maintaining *all* muscular activity—with a particular sensitivity to cardiac muscle—through its role in the sodium-potassium pump

2. Along with sodium, potassium maintains acid–base balance as it exchanges for hydrogen.

3. It also is required for all metabolic processes, including:

   a. Carbohydrate metabolism
   b. Glycogen synthesis
   c. Protein synthesis

D. Regulation

1. Potassium is regulated by:

   a. Renal mechanisms
   b. Extrarenal mechanisms

2. *Renal mechanisms* include:

   a. Glomerular filtration
   b. Tubular reabsorption
   c. Tubular secretion
   d. Renin-aldosterone mechanism
   e. Plasma protein regulation
   f. Sodium regulation
   g. Metabolic acidosis

3. In *glomerular filtration*, blood is filtered in the glomerulus, where the filtered load enters the proximal tubule.

4. In *tubular reabsorption*:

   a. The epithelial cells of the proximal tubule reabsorb approximately 65% of the filtered potassium through active transport.
   b. The thick portion of the ascending limb of Henle's loop reabsorbs about 27%, leaving 8% of the original filtered load to enter the distal tubules.
   c. The distal and collecting tubules absorb a very slight amount of potassium, but potassium secretion occurs here.

5. In *tubular secretion*, potassium moves from the blood to the tubular lumen:

   a. The amount of potassium secretion is determined by the need for potassium elimination, which is influenced by the serum concentration level.

      b. Potassium is exchanged for hydrogen to maintain electrical neutrality across the cell membrane.

      c. Because potassium and sodium must exchange for balance, the sodium concentration and the presence of aldosterone will increase absorption of sodium from the tubules to the serum, making potassium exchange the other way (eg, be excreted) to achieve balance.

6. The distal tubule's secretory function provides evidence of why hyperkalemia is consistent with tubular defects seen in various forms of acute and chronic renal failure.

7. During end-stage renal disease, glomerular filtration or tubular reabsorption and secretion fail.

8. The *renin-aldosterone mechanism,* which is mediated by angiotensin, brings a supply of aldosterone to the distal tubule and affects potassium levels:

      a. Aldosterone in the tubule causes reabsorption of sodium, which in turn causes potassium to move in the opposite direction from the blood into the tubule for secretions.

      b. Aldosterone also stimulates potassium uptake in the proximal tubule, increasing the concentration of peritubular potassium. This enhances passive diffusion of potassium into the tubular lumen for excretion when it arrives in the distal tubule. This mechanism is targeted during administration of certain medications, such as Aldactone.

9. *Plasma protein* levels regulate potassium because an increase in plasma protein concentration causes a subsequent rise in the rate of potassium transport into the tubular lumen. This results from an increase in ICF electrical negativity that pulls potassium into the tubular cells and then into the tubular lumen.

10. *Sodium regulation* affects potassium levels:

      a. When the amount of sodium entering the distal tubule increases, the rate of sodium reabsorption by the distal end of the tubules and collecting ducts also increases.

      b. As a result, potassium secretion, which normally moves in the opposite direction of sodium reabsorption by the distal end of the tubules and collecting ducts, also is increased.

      c. The sodium delivery to the distal tubule fosters potassium secretion by increasing the transmembrane electrical difference.

      d. Situations that contribute to natriuresis (sodium elimination) increase potassium elimination and increase the osmotic load that exists when a large water supply is present.

      e. The larger the osmotic load delivered to the proximal tubule, the less potassium reabsorbed at this point, which makes more available for elimination.

11. *Metabolic acidosis* affects potassium levels as it is exchanged for hydrogen:

a. During metabolic acidosis, hydrogen levels rise, then hydrogen moves to the ICF and potassium moves out of the ICF to restore electrical neutrality.

b. As a result, the ICF concentration of potassium in the distal tubule is diminished.

c. Additional bicarbonate wasting provides accelerated distal delivery of the anion, increasing potassium secretion in another attempt to maintain electrical neutrality.

12. *Extrarenal mechanisms* that affect potassium regulation include:
    a. GI system
    b. Fluid shifts
    c. Hydration

13. In the *GI system*, the mucosa of the large bowel is readily responsive to some of the same stimulators of kaliuresis (potassium excretion):
    a. Mineralocorticoid activity causes sodium reabsorption and potassium elimination from the same mechanism that occurs in the kidney.
    b. Accelerated bowel elimination of potassium is an important adaptive mechanism. (For this reason, patients undergoing bowel surgery or those with large amounts of GI drainage must be watched closely for dropping potassium levels.)

14. Potassium levels are sensitive to hormonal fluctuations and any conditions that could cause *fluid shifts*, including:
    a. Adrenocorticotropic hormone (ACTH) secretion: ACTH is secreted from the anterior pituitary to stimulate steroid secretion from the adrenal glands, making aldosterone levels dependent on ACTH levels. In the presence of aldosterone, sodium is retained and potassium is excreted. Potassium levels drop when ACTH levels rise due to the relationship between ACTH and aldosterone. Potassium levels rise as ACTH and aldosterone levels drop, because sodium is eliminated rather than reabsorbed.
    b. Increased glucose levels: As glucose levels rise, potassium is transported into the cells. As glucose levels drop, potassium leaves the cell.

15. *Hydration* affects potassium levels in two ways:
    a. Increased body water (hypervolemia) can dilute potassium, causing levels to drop.
    b. Dehydration (hypovolemia) causes an increase in potassium concentration, resulting in higher serum levels.

II. Potassium deficiency: Hypokalemia

A. Description: Serum potassium level below 3.5 mEq/L

B. Etiology

1. Potassium loss, such as from:
   a. Prolonged diuretic therapy (because potassium follows water and sodium across the tubular membrane)

      b. Prolonged vomiting, diarrhea, laxative abuse, or nasogastric suctioning (because bile and GI secretions are rich in potassium)

      c. Severe diaphoresis

      d. Renal tubule defects (eg, renal tubular acidosis)

      e. Excessive removal of potassium during peritoneal dialysis or hemodialysis

  2. Inadequate intake or absorption due to:

      a. Anorexia

      b. Acute alcoholism

  3. Fluid and electrolyte shifts due to:

      a. Administration of potassium-deficient hyperalimentation solutions

      b. Administration of hypertonic glucose solutions (because potassium may shift from ECF to ICF)

      c. Presence of excessive amounts of exogenous or endogenous insulin (because insulin acts as a carrier molecule, aiding intracellular transport of potassium)

      d. Presence of excessive steroid hormones (because corticosteroid levels influence sodium retention and reciprocal potassium excretion)

      e. Lowered levels of extracellular hydrogen (such as occurs in metabolic alkalosis)

      f. Hyperaldosteronism (which causes excessive absorption of sodium in the proximal tubules, accounting for accelerated excretion of potassium)

C. Assessment findings

  1. Clinical manifestations may include vomiting or diarrhea; however, these symptoms may be the cause of hypokalemia.

  2. Because potassium is required for normal musculoskeletal contractions, alterations will affect the musculoskeletal system. Symptoms may include:

      a. Muscle weakness and cramps

      b. Hyporeflexia

      c. Paresthesias

      d. Decreased bowel motility (which could develop into paralytic ileus)

      e. Hypotension

      f. Cardiac dysrhythmia

      g. Drowsiness, lethargy, coma

  3. Laboratory results reveal:

      a. Serum potassium level below 3.5 mEq/L

      b. pH elevated above 7.45

      c. Decreased serum bicarbonate level

      d. Elevated glucose level (possible)

  4. Another diagnostic cue is electrocardiogram (EKG) changes; as potassium levels drop, the EKG will gradually reveal ST segment depression, flattened T waves, and U waves that may be hidden on the T waves (Fig. 6–1).

D. **Potential nursing diagnoses**

1. Decreased Cardiac Output
2. High Risk for Injury

E. **Interventions**

1. Prevent hypokalemia and ensure early detection by identifying high-risk patients (eg, those who have anorexia, diarrhea, or nausea and vomiting) and providing appropriate patient education.
2. Teach patients receiving diuretic therapy at home about hypokalemia and how to manage it.
3. Be aware that in patients receiving digitalis, digitalis toxicity may occur (especially if Lasix is administered concurrently).
4. Monitor intake and output, keeping in mind that urine contains potassium.
5. Replace potassium through dietary intervention (eg, encourage the patient to eat or drink citrus fruits and juices).
6. Administer oral potassium replacements, as ordered; be aware that these can irritate the GI mucosa, so give them with water.
7. When adding potassium to a liter of IV solution:
   a. Be sure the drip rate is adjusted so that replacement does not occur too quickly.

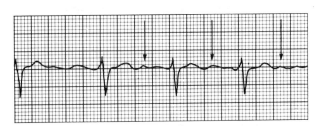

A

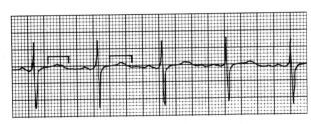

B

FIGURE 6–1.
(A) Presence of U waves (hypokalemia). **(B)** Fusion of T and U waves (hypokalemia).

      b.   Be aware that the insertion site may become reddened and painfully irritated.

      c.   Be sure to mix the solution thoroughly, or the patient may inadvertently receive a potassium bolus.

      d.   Keep in mind that rapid administration of potassium can cause sudden hyperkalemia, which can cause cardiac arrest.

  8. For life-threatening hypokalemia:

      a.   Replace potassium more rapidly by adding 10 mEq of potassium chloride to 100 mL of IV solution and infusing over 1 hour using an infusion pump.

      b.   Use *extreme caution*, and *never administer potassium by IV push method*, which could cause death.

      c.   Institute cardiac monitoring.

  9. Monitor vital signs.

  10. Monitor serum potassium levels.

  11. Monitor for signs of other associated electrolyte disorders (eg, alkalosis).

F. **Evaluation**

  1. Serum potassium level returns to a range between 3.5 and 5.0 mEq/L.

  2. The patient's cardiac output is normal.

  3. The patient is free from injury.

III. Potassium excess: Hyperkalemia

A. **Description: Serum potassium level above 5.0 mEq/L**

B. **Etiology**

  1. Potassium intake in excess of potassium excretion, such as from:

      a.   IV replacement potassium

      b.   Potassium-rich hyperalimentation solutions

      c.   Use of potassium replacements

      d.   Excessive use of salt substitutes

  2. Poor potassium elimination due to:

      a.   Kidney failure (in which the tubules are unable to balance potassium)

      b.   Bowel obstruction

      c.   Use of potassium-sparing diuretics (spironolactone)

  3. Electrolyte shifts in which a cation must leave the intracellular space, such as in:

      a.   Metabolic acidosis: Hydrogen enters the cell in exchange for potassium, which leaves the cell and enters the ECF.

      b.   Hyponatremia: When sodium is lost, potassium will move in the opposite direction and be retained.

  4. Cell lysis: In burns, trauma, cancer chemotherapy, or any condition causing great cell damage, potassium is released into the serum.

C. Assessment findings

1. Symptoms of hyperkalemia may be life-threatening.
2. Because potassium is required for normal nerve and muscle contractions, hyperkalemia affects the musculoskeletal system, smooth muscle function, and nerve cell function; symptoms may include:
   a. Confusion
   b. Paresthesia
   c. Abdominal cramps with possible diarrhea
   d. Muscle paralysis
3. Because potassium is required for normal cardiac functioning, patients with hyperkalemia may present with life-threatening arrhythmias. As potassium levels rise, EKG changes worsen and include prolonged P-R interval, wide QRS complex, and full T waves (which may be tented). Eventually, these changes lead to cardiac arrest (Fig. 6–2).

D. Potential nursing diagnoses

1. Decreased Cardiac Output
2. High Risk for Injury
3. Immobility

E. Interventions

1. Identify high-risk patients (eg, those receiving potassium-sparing diuretics, potassium supplements, or IV potassium and those with renal failure and metabolic acidosis).
2. Check the patient's urine output and potassium levels before administering any medication containing potassium.
3. Provide cardiac monitoring.
4. If hyperkalemia is excessive, prepare the patient for administration of Kayexelate, a glucose and insulin drip, or hemodialysis, as ordered.
5. Administer sodium bicarbonate if ordered; be sure to administer this *with caution* because it can cause calcium levels to drop.
6. Monitor intake and output.

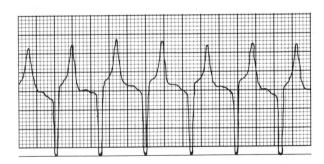

FIGURE 6–2.
Hyperkalemia and the presence of peaked T waves.

F. Evaluation

 1. Serum potassium level returns to a range between 3.5 and 5.0 mEq/L.
 2. The patient remains free of symptoms.
 3. Cardiac output is not decreased.
 4. The patient is mobile and free from injury.

Bibliography

Alspach, J. G. (1991). *Core curriculum for critical care nursing* (4th ed.). Philadelphia: W.B. Saunders.

Brunner, L. S., & Suddarth, D. S. (1992). *Textbook of medical-surgical nursing* (7th ed.). Philadelphia: J.B. Lippincott.

Guyton, A. (1991). *Textbook of medical physiology* (8th ed.). Philadelphia: W.B. Saunders.

McCance, K. L., & Huether, S. E. (1994). *Pathophysiology: The biologic basis for disease in adults and children* (2nd ed.). St. Louis: Mosby–Year Book.

Metheny, N. (1992). *Fluid and electrolyte balance: Nursing considerations* (2nd ed.). Philadelphia: J.B. Lippincott.

STUDY QUESTIONS

1. When assessing a patient for potassium deficits, the nurse is aware that normal serum potassium level ranges from:
   a. 1.5 to 3.5 mEq/dl
   b. 2.5 to 4.5 mEq/dl
   c. 3.5 to 5.0 mEq/dl
   d. 4.0 to 7.5 mEq/dl

2. A patient who is on Lasix therapy asks the nurse about potassium-rich foods; which of the following foods would the nurse recommend?
   a. oranges
   b. apples
   c. pears
   d. peaches

3. Which of the following interventions would the nurse undertake for a patient receiving IV replacement of potassium?
   a. Assess level of consciousness.
   b. Monitor pulse.
   c. Monitor blood pressure.
   d. Assess the IV site.

4. Conditions that increase natriuresis result in:
   a. increased osmotic load and increased potassium excretion
   b. decreased osmotic load and decreased potassium excretion
   c. increased osmotic load and decreased potassium excretion
   d. decreased osmotic load and increased potassium excretion

5. Which of the following symptoms is *not* associated with hypokalemia?
   a. muscle cramps
   b. U waves on EKG
   c. paresthesia
   d. hyperreflexia

6. When assessing a patient for hyperkalemia, the nurse would *not* expect to assess:
   a. U waves on EKG
   b. paresthesia
   c. muscle paralysis
   d. tented T waves on EKG

7. Before administering any medication containing potassium, an important nursing intervention is to check the patient's:
   a. EKG
   b. pulse
   c. blood pressure
   d. urine output

8. Metabolic acidosis results in which of the following electrolyte shifts?
   a. Hydrogen ions are excreted with potassium and sodium.
   b. Hydrogen ions enter the ECF and potassium moves to the ICF.
   c. Hydrogen ions enter the cells and potassium moves to the ECF.
   d. Bicarbonate enters the cells in exchange for potassium ions.

ANSWER KEY

1. *Correct response: c*
   Normal serum potassium level ranges
   from 3.5 to 5.0 mEq/dl.
   a, b, and d. Serum potassium level
   below 3.5 is hypokalemia; above
   5.0, hyperkalemia.
   Knowledge/Health Promotion/Assessment

2. *Correct response: a*
   Citrus fruits, vegetables, chocolate, and
   licorice are good sources of potassium.
   b, c, and d. These responses are incorrect.
   Knowledge/Safe Care/Analysis

3. *Correct response: d*
   Potassium supplements are irritating, so
   careful IV site assessment is necessary.
   a, b and c. These interventions are
   not related to IV administration of
   potassium.
   *Comprehension/Safe
   Care/Implementation*

4. *Correct response: a*
   Conditions associated with natriuresis
   increase osmotic load and potassium
   excretion.
   b, c and d. These responses are incorrect.
   Analysis/Physiologic/Assessment

5. *Correct response: d*
   Hyporeflexia, not hyperreflexia, is a
   symptom of hypokalemia.

   a, b and c. Muscle cramps, U waves
   on the EKG, and paresthesia are additional symptoms of hypokalemia.
   Knowledge/Physiologic/Assessment

6. *Correct response: a*
   U waves on EKG indicate hypokalemia.
   b, c and d. Paresthesia, muscle paralysis, and tented T waves are symptoms of hyperkalemia.
   Knowledge/Safe Care/Assessment

7. *Correct response: d*
   Since kidney failure is an etiology of hyperkalemia, it is important that the
   nurse determine the patient's urine output before administering medications
   containing potassium.
   a, b, and c. These are important parameters to assess, but are not specific to potassium.
   Knowledge/Safe Care/Implementation

8. *Correct response: c*
   In metabolic acidosis, hydrogen ions
   enter the cells in exchange for potassium, which then leaves the cells and
   enters the ECF.
   a, b, and d. These are electrolyte shifts
   that are not associated with metabolic acidosis.
   Knowledge/Safe Care/NA

Chloride: Normal
and Altered Balance

I. Normal balance
A. Description
   1. Chloride is the major anion in extracellular fluid (ECF).
   2. Normal values: Serum chloride levels range from 95 to 108 mEq/L.

B. Supply and sources
   1. Chloride is taken in through the diet, especially from foods rich in salt.
   2. It is found in combination with sodium in the blood as sodium chloride (NaCl).
   3. It is found in combination with hydrogen in the stomach as hydrogen chloride (HCl).

C. Functions
   1. Works with sodium to maintain serum osmolarity
   2. Maintains the balance of cations in the intracellular fluid (ICF) and ECF.
   3. Participates in maintaining acid–base balance through a mechanism called the chloride shift:

a. Chloride shifts into and out of red blood cells in exchange for bicarbonate to maintain acid–base balance (Fig. 7–1).

b. As part of maintaining acid–base balance, carbonic acid (H_2CO_3), which is formed in the red blood cells (RBCs), separates into H and HCO_3.

c. The hydrogen ion attaches to hemoglobin, and the HCO_3 is free to leave the RBCs and circulate in the plasma; if this were to occur, there would be an excess of HCO_3 in the plasma.

d. However, as HCO_3 diffuses out of the RBCs and into the plasma, chloride shifts into the RBCs to maintain electrical neutrality in the RBCs.

e. A special protein (known as the bicarbonate-chloride carrier protein) shifts these two electrolytes back and forth into and out of the RBCs.

D. Regulation

1. Chloride is regulated by renal and extrarenal mechanisms.

2. *Renal regulation:*

   a. Plasma concentration of chloride is regulated by the kidneys through reabsorption and is equal to the amount of chloride filtered through the glomerulus.

   b. Chloride reabsorption depends on sodium reabsorption, which is regulated by aldosterone in the distal tubule and collecting ducts. Any alteration in sodium reabsorption will secondarily affect the chloride level.

   c. Chloride is excreted in the urine; the amount excreted is related to the amount taken in through the diet or intravenous infusion or to the amount needed by the body.

3. *Extrarenal regulation:*

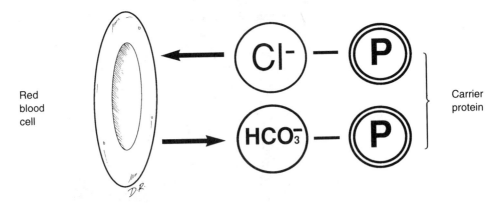

FIGURE 7–1.
The chloride shift. A special carrier protein exchanges chloride and bicarbonate ions into and out of the red blood cells.

      a. Chloride is absorbed in the bowel (mainly the duodenum and jejunum) as it passively follows sodium to maintain electrical neutrality across the bowel wall.

      b. Chloride also is actively absorbed in the ileum and large intestine by a specialized transport mechanism.

      c. In this transport mechanism, a number of chloride ions are reabsorbed for an equal number of secreted bicarbonate ions; bicarbonate moves directly from the serum into the bowel and is exchanged for chloride ions to maintain electrical neutrality.

      d. This mechanism allows bicarbonate to neutralize acids created by intestinal bacteria.

II. Chloride deficiency: Hypochloremia

A. Description

1. Hypochloremia is a condition in which the serum chloride level is below 95 mEq/L.

2. When chloride concentrations drop below 95 mEq/L, bicarbonate reabsorption increases proportionally, causing metabolic alkalosis.

3. The increase in bicarbonate is usually accompanied by a shift of intercellular hydrogen out of the cell and potassium into the cell, causing hypokalemia.

B. Etiology

1. Excessive losses through the GI system, such as from:
   a. Vomiting
   b. Nasogastric suctioning
   c. Irrigation

2. Sodium deficits related to restricted intake or losses through diuretics

3. Losses through the urine due to:
   a. Diuretic therapy (which can alter various electrolyte levels)
   b. Chloriduria (excessive excretion of chloride in the urine); this condition, which usually results from increased chloride intake, commonly occurs in patients with Bartter's syndrome who are receiving potassium chloride to treat hypokalemia. Another possible cause of chloriduria is a defect of sodium reabsorption in the renal tubules.

4. Chloridorrhea, a congenital disorder that presents with frequent loose stools, resulting in increased loss of hydrochloric acid and increased renal hydrogen excretion

5. Excessive water within the body (eg, due to overinfusion of hypotonic solutions or excessive water intake); known as dilutional hypochloremia

C. Assessment findings

1. No specific symptoms are associated with hypochloremia, which

usually occurs secondary to other pathophysiologic processes (eg, cystic fibrosis) along with changes in other electrolytes.

    2. Laboratory tests reveal serum chloride level below 95 mEq/L.

D. Potential nursing diagnoses

    1. High Risk for Injury

    2. Fluid Volume Excess

E. Interventions

    1. Assist in achieving the treatment objective of restoring the chloride level within the range of 95 to 108 mEq/L.

    2. Institute measures to manage the underlying disorder.

    3. Replace fluids, as ordered, to restore and maintain serum osmolarity.

    4. Replace electrolytes as needed to maintain acid–base balance.

    5. Monitor serum electrolytes.

F. Evaluation

    1. Serum chloride level returns to a range between 95 and 108 mEq/L.

    2. Serum electrolyte levels remain in normal ranges.

    3. The underlying disorder is corrected.

    4. The patient's fluid volume is normal.

    5. The patient is free from injury.

III. Chloride excess: Hyperchloremia

A. Description: Serum chloride level above 108 mEq/L.

B. Etiology

    1. Sodium excess (hypernatremia)

    2. Bicarbonate deficit (metabolic acidosis)

C. Assessment findings

    1. No specific symptoms are associated with hyperchloremia, which usually occurs secondary to other electrolyte disorders.

    2. Hyperchloremia can occur with hypernatremia or metabolic acidosis.

    3. Laboratory tests reveal serum chloride level above 108 mEq/L.

D. Potential nursing diagnoses vary with coexisting disorder.

    1. Fluid Volume Deficit

    2. High Risk for Injury

E. Interventions

    1. Identify patient at risk, especially those using diuretics.

    2. Institute measures to manage the underlying disorder.

    3. Monitor serum electrolytes.

    4. Monitor fluid intake and output.

    5. Monitor urinary concentration of chloride.

    6. Monitor the patient's ingestion of chloride from sources such as table salt, fruit, vegetables, and excess water intake.

F. **Evaluation**
1. Serum chloride level returns to a range between 95 and 108 mEq/L.
2. Serum electrolyte levels remain in normal ranges.
3. The underlying disorder is corrected.
4. The patient's fluid volume is normal.
5. The patient is free of injury.

Bibliography

Gröer, M. (1981). *Physiology and pathophysiology of the body fluids.* St. Louis: C.V. Mosby.

Carroll, H., & Oh, M. (1989). *Water, electrolyte and acid-base metabolism* (2nd ed.). Philadelphia: J.B. Lippincott.

McCance, K., & Huether, S. (1990). *Pathophysiology: The biologic basis for disease in adults and children.* St. Louis: C.V. Mosby.

Byrne, J., Saxton, D., Pelikan, P., & Nugent, P. (1986). *Laboratory tests: Implications for nursing care* (2nd ed.). California: Addison-Wesley Publishing.

STUDY QUESTIONS

1. On admission, a patient's serum chloride level is 90 mEq/L. The nurse interprets this as:
   a. low
   b. high
   c. within the normal range
   d. unable to be interpreted

2. Chloride is a major anion found in the extracellular fluid (ECF); chloride levels fluctuate in response to:
   a. H_2O levels
   b. potassium levels
   c. HCO_3 levels
   d. hemoglobin levels

3. Hypochloremia may be associated with all of the following *except:*
   a. vomiting
   b. decreased water intake
   c. diuretic therapy
   d. fistula drainage

4. When assessing a patient for hyperchloremia, the nurse would expect to find which of the following concurrent conditions?
   a. metabolic alkalosis
   b. hyponatremia
   c. hypernatremia
   d. excessive bicarbonate

5. Chloridorrhea is a congenital disorder typically resulting in:
   a. decreased HCO_3 production
   b. excessive potassium
   c. excessive HCL loss
   d. decreased renal hydrogen excretion

6. When caring for a patient with gastrointestinal disease, the nurse is aware that which of the following therapies might cause chloride loss?
   a. retention enemas
   b. cathartics
   c. nasogastric suctioning
   d. nasogastric tube feeding

7. Hypochloremia is associated with which of the following electrolyte disorders?
   a. hyperkalemia
   b. hyponatremia
   c. hypermagnesemia
   d. hyperphosphatemia

8. Chloride shift exchanges chloride for which of the following electrolytes?
   a. sodium
   b. potassium
   c. bicarbonate
   d. hydrogen

ANSWER KEY

1. **Correct response: a**
   Serum chloride level below 95 mEq/L is low, indicating hypochloremia.
   b. Serum chloride level above 108 mEq/L is high, indicating hyperchloremia.
   c. Normal serum chloride levels range from 95 to 108 mEq/L.
   d. This response is incorrect.
   Analysis/Physiologic/Assessment

2. **Correct response: c**
   ECF chloride levels fluctuate with levels of bicarbonate (HCO_3); as HCO_3 levels increase, chloride levels decrease.
   a, b, and d. These responses are incorrect.
   Analysis/Physiologic/Assessment

3. **Correct response: b**
   Dilutional hypochloremia may be seen in states of excessive, not decreased water intake.
   a, c, and d. Hypochloremia is associated with vomiting, diuretic therapy, and fistula drainage.
   Analysis/Physiologic/Assessment

4. **Correct response: c**
   Greater than normal amounts of chloride can be expected with hypernatremia.
   a. Metabolic acidosis, not alkalosis, is present.
   b. Hypernatremia, not hyponatremia, is present
   d. Decreased, not excessive HCO_3, is present.
   Analysis/Physiologic/Analysis

5. **Correct response: c**
   Chloridorrhea presents with frequent loose stools, resulting in increased loss of HCl.
   a, b, and d. Chloridorrhea results in increased HCO_3 production, decreased potassium, and increased renal hydrogen excretion.
   Comprehension/Physiologic/Assessment

6. **Correct response: c**
   Nasogastric suctioning may result in excessive chloride loss, since gastric fluid is rich in chlorides.
   a, b and d. These therapies are not related to loss of any electrolytes.
   Application/Safe Care/Planning

7. **Correct response: b**
   Hypochloremia is associated with sodium deficits related to restricted intake or losses through diuretics.
   a, c, and d. These responses are incorrect.
   Comprehension/Physiologic/Assessment

8. **Correct response: c**
   Chloride exchanges for bicarbonate in the red blood cells, helping to maintain acid–base balance. When the hydrogen ion attaches to hemoglobin, bicarbonate exits and chloride shifts in to maintain electrical neutrality.
   a, b and d. These electrolytes do not exchange for chloride during the chloride shift.
   Comprehension/Physiologic/Analysis

Calcium: Normal and Altered Balance

I. Normal balance

A. Description

1. Calcium is a major cation; total body content is about 1200 g.
2. Normal serum calcium level ranges from 8.5 to 10.5 mg/dL.
3. Calcium is regulated closely with magnesium and phosphorus.

B. Supply and sources

1. Most of the total body calcium is bound to bone.
2. Calcium that is not bound to bone is either bound to plasma protein or is ionized.
3. Ionized calcium performs vital metabolic functions.
4. Calcium is taken in through the diet; recommended daily calcium intake is 800 mg.
5. Abnormal routes of calcium intake include intravenous (IV) administration or hyperalimentation.

C. Functions

1. Calcium is mobilized through a complicated metabolic pathway that involves the endocrine, renal, and gastrointestinal (GI) systems.

Paradiso, C: *Lippincott's Review Series: Fluids and Electrolytes* © 1995 J. B. Lippincott Company

2. Calcium that is bound to bone contributes to bone and tooth rigidity and strength.
3. Some calcium is bound to protein, so abnormal calcium levels are analyzed in relation to proteins.
4. Ionized calcium is required as an enzymatic cofactor for blood clotting.
5. Calcium also is:
   a. Partially responsible for maintaining cell membrane structure and function
   b. Required for neuromuscular conduction by its participation in the sodium-potassium pump
   c. Required for cardiac contraction
   d. Required for hormonal secretions

D. Regulation
   1. *GI regulation*:
      a. Calcium is absorbed in the GI tract.
      b. Vitamin D in its biologically active form, known as 1,25-dihydroxycholecalciferol (1,25 DHC), is required for the absorption of calcium; this conversion of vitamin D occurs in the kidneys.
   2. *Renal regulation*:
      a. Calcium is filtered in the glomerulus and reabsorbed in the tubules.
      b. When excessive calcium is present, it may precipitate to form stones.
   3. *Endocrine regulation*:
      a. The parathyroid gland responds to low plasma calcium by releasing parathyroid hormone (PTH).
      b. PTH in turn stimulates the release of calcium from bone into the serum to bring serum levels to normal (Fig. 8–1); over many years, this depletes the bone, contributing to osteoporosis.
      c. However, if serum phosphorus levels are higher than normal, the calcium will bind with the phosphorus.
      d. This binding of calcium and phosphorus, known as calcium phosphate or the phosphate product, can be detrimental; if the calcium phosphate product exceeds 70 mEq/L. Soft-tissue calcification of the eyes, blood vessels, and cardiac conduction system may occur.
      e. Calcitonin, a thyroid hormone, moves calcium from plasma to bone when serum levels rise.

II. Calcium deficiency: Hypocalcemia
   A. Description: Serum calcium level below 8.5 mg/dL
   B. Etiology
      1. Inadequate intake or absorption of calcium due to:

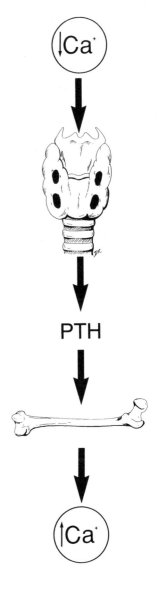

FIGURE 8–1.
PTH and calcium. Decreasing serum calcium levels pull calcium out of bone into serum through the action of PTH.

      a. Anorexia
      b. Acute or chronic renal failure (in these conditions 1,25 DHC is not produced)
      c. Vitamin D deficiency
      d. Inadequate exposure to ultraviolet light, which hinders conversion of vitamin D to its active form
  2. Excessive elimination or excretion (eg, as occurs in patients on large doses of Lasix)
  3. Low PTH levels, which reduce calcium absorption
  4. Electrolyte shifts due to:

a. Hypoparathyroidism, which reduces levels of PTH
b. Renal failure, which causes hyperphosphatemia; this imbalance reduces serum calcium as the excessive phosphorus binds with ionized calcium.

5. Excessive administration of HCO_3, because the HCO_3 binds with ionized calcium (possible cause)

C. **Assessment findings**

1. Because calcium is a critical part of neuromuscular contraction, falling calcium levels affect the contraction of smooth, skeletal, and cardiac muscles; symptoms may include:
   a. Muscle cramps in arms and legs
   b. Muscle spasms (spasms in bronchial and laryngeal muscles are particularly dangerous)
   c. Cardiac dysrhythmias (eg, prolonged Q-T interval) (Fig. 8–2);
2. Calcium also is a critical part of nerve cell conduction. Low plasma calcium levels make nerve cells more excitable. This occurs because a lack of calcium causes increased neural permeability to sodium. Manifestations include:
   a. Hyperactive deep-tendon reflexes
   b. Paresthesia of extremities
   c. Positive Chvostek's and Trousseau's signs
   d. Confusion
   e. Moodiness and anxiety
   f. Hypocalcemic tetany and seizures (possible dangerous sequelae)
   g. Electrocardiogram changes
3. Because calcium is needed for normal blood clotting, symptoms associated with excessive bleeding may occur; these can include:
   a. Easy bruising and petechiae
   b. Excessive bleeding when cut
4. Laboratory tests reveal:

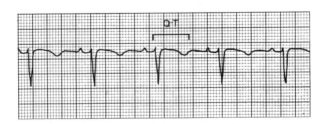

FIGURE 8–2.
Prolonged Q-T interval (hypocalcemia). For this heart rate of 70 beats/minute, the Q-T interval should be between 0.31 and 0.38 seconds. This patient's Q-T interval measures 0.50 seconds because his serum calcium level is 5.4 mg/dL. (Normal serum calcium is 8.5–10.5 mg/dL).

       a. Serum calcium levels below 8.5 mg/dL

       b. Hyperphosphatemia (because decreased calcium levels result in increased phosphorus levels)

       c. Hypomagnesemia or hypoalbuminemia (may be present)

       d. Prolonged prothrombin time and partial thromboplastin time (because calcium is required for blood clotting)

D. Potential nursing diagnoses

    1. Ineffective Breathing Patterns related to altered calcium

    2. Decreased Cardiac Output

    3. High Risk for Injury

E. Interventions

    1. Identify patients at risk for hypocalcemia (eg, those who have had thyroidectomy and those with GI or renal disorders).

    2. Institute cardiac monitoring, and secure precautions if the patient's calcium level is dangerously low.

    3. Assist in achieving the treatment objective of restoring the calcium level within a range between 8.5 and 10.5 mg/dL.

    4. For moderate loss:

       a. Give oral supplements, as ordered, with vitamin D. Be aware that if hyperphosphatemia is present, phosphate supplements also must be given because there is a danger that the calcium supplement will bind with the phosphorus and create an excess calcium phosphate product.

       b. Provide nutritional counseling if hypocalcemia is due to dietary deficiency.

       c. Instruct the patient that exercise enhances calcium mobilization from bone and will replenish plasma calcium levels.

    5. For dangerously low levels:

       a. Replace calcium with IV calcium gluconate as ordered. Be aware that a large vein is needed for IV calcium replacement and that infiltration can cause sloughing.

       b. Institute cardiac monitoring.

       c. Administer calcium *with caution* to patients on digoxin, because it sensitizes the heart to digoxin.

F. Evaluation

    1. Serum calcium level returns to a range between 8.5 and 10.5 mg/dL.

    2. The patient's breathing patterns are normal.

    3. The patient experiences no bleeding.

    4. The patient's cardiac output is normal.

    5. The patient is free from injury.

III. Calcium excess: Hypercalcemia

A. Description: serum calcium level above 10.5 mg/dL

B. Etiology

    1. Excessive calcium intake or absorption, such as from:•

      a.   Overzealous use of calcium supplements
      b.   Increased vitamin D intake
      c.   Altered GI metabolism
      d.   Medications (eg, calcium-containing antacids and phosphate binding gels)

2. Metabolic conditions, such as:
      a.   Hyperparathyroidism, which accelerates PTH effects on bone and removes bound calcium to the serum
      b.   Renal tubule disorders, which reduce the efficiency of renal electrolyte regulation
      c.   Hypophosphatemia (because phosphorus and calcium have an inversely reciprocal relationship)
      d.   Thyrotoxicosis, which accelerates calcitonin secretion
      e.   Bone disorders (eg, cancers and metastatic lesions, accelerated bone metabolism)
      f.   Immobility, which alters bone metabolism

C. **Assessment findings**
   1. Symptom severity increases as the calcium level rises.
   2. Rising calcium level affects the skeletal, smooth, and cardiac muscles; manifestations may include:
      a.   Decreased peristalsis, resulting in constipation
      b.   Muscle weakness or flaccidity
      c.   Cardiac dysrhythmias, reflected in shortened Q-T interval (Fig. 8–3)
   3. Neurologic manifestations occur because calcium affects conduction across nerve cells; symptoms may include:
      a.   Confusion
      b.   Personality changes
      c.   Altered level of consciousness
      d.   Coma
   4. Because calcium plays a role in many metabolic processes, manifestations may occur in other systems; these include:
      a.   Urinary calculi (may be present as calcium precipitates in the kidney)

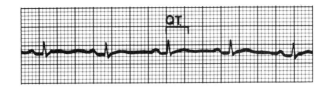

FIGURE 8–3.
Shortened Q-T interval (hypercalcemia). The normal Q-T interval for the above heart rate of 88 beats/minute is 0.28 second to 0.36 second. This patient's serum calcium level is 12.1 mg/dL, and the Q-T interval measures 0.24 second.

b. GI alterations (eg, anorexia, thirst, nausea, and vomiting)
c. Pathologic fractures (can result when calcium leaves the bone)
d. Soft-tissue calcification
5. Laboratory and diagnostic tests reveal:
a. Serum calcium level above 10.5 mg/dL
b. Bone changes and reduced bone density

D. Potential nursing diagnoses
1. Decreased Cardiac Output
2. High Risk for Injury

E. Interventions
1. Institute measures to prevent hypercalcemia:
a. Recognize high-risk patients, and instruct them to avoid calcium-rich foods.
b. Ambulate patients as early as possible.
2. Institute measures to eliminate excess calcium:
a. Administer loop diuretics (eg, Lasix) as ordered to facilitate calcium removal.
b. Administer IV normal saline as ordered to foster diuresis and subsequent calcium elimination.
3. Administer calcitonin as ordered to lower serum calcium levels.
4. Monitor electrolyte status.

F. Evaluation
1. Serum calcium level returns to normal range.
2. The patient's cardiac output is normal.
3. The patient is free from injury.

Bibliography

Alspach, J. G. (1991). *Core curriculum for critical care nursing* (4th ed.). Philadelphia: W.B. Saunders.

Brunner, L. S., & Suddarth, D. S. (1992). *Textbook of medical-surgical nursing* (7th ed.). Philadelphia: J.B. Lippincott.

Guyton, A. (1991). *Textbook of medical physiology* (8th ed.). Philadelphia: W.B. Saunders.

McCance, K. L., & Huether, S. E. (1994). *Pathophysiology: The biologic basis for disease in adults and children* (2nd ed.). St. Louis: Mosby–Year Book.

Metheny, N. (1992). *Fluid and electrolyte balance: Nursing considerations* (2nd ed.). Philadelphia: J.B. Lippincott.

STUDY QUESTIONS

1. Normal serum calcium levels are:
   a. 800 mg
   b. 1200 mg
   c. 8.5 to 10.5 mg/dl
   d. 2.5 to 4.5 mg/dl

2. Serum calcium levels rise with metastatic bone lesions because of:
   a. hyperphosphatemia
   b. osteoporosis
   c. chemotherapy
   d. accelerated bone metabolism

3. When assessing a patient for hypocalcemia, the nurse would *not* expect to find:
   a. hyperactive deep tendon reflexes
   b. prolonged Q-T interval on EKG
   c. muscle weakness
   d. decreased peristalsis

4. When educating a patient about foods high in calcium, the nurse would recommend:
   a. canned fish
   b. coffee
   c. dry beans
   d. meat

5. Nursing interventions for a patient with hypocalcemia may include:
   a. encouraging bedrest
   b. administering IV calcium gluconate
   c. administering calcitonin
   d. using loop diuretics

6. When caring for a patient with hypercalcemia, the nurse should plan to administer which of the following drugs?
   a. Inderal
   b. bicarbonate
   c. Lasix
   d. mannitol

7. The most dangerous sequela of hypercalcemia is:
   a. constipation
   b. muscle weakness
   c. dyspnea
   d. dysrhythmias

8. Which one of the following metabolic conditions places a patient at high risk for hypercalcemia?
   a. myxedema
   b. exercise
   c. hyperphosphatemia
   d. hyperparathyroidism

ANSWER KEY

1. ***Correct response: c***
Normal calcium level ranges from 8.5 to 10.5 mg/dl.
a, b, and d. These responses are incorrect.
Knowledge/Physiologic/Assessment

2. ***Correct response: d***
Bone cancers and metastatic lesions result in hypercalcemia because of accelerated bone metabolism, which causes calcium to be released from the bone to the blood.
a. Hyperphosphatemia would result in hypocalcemia.
b and c. These responses are incorrect.
Analysis/Physiologic/Analysis

3. ***Correct response: d***
Decreased peristalsis resulting in constipation is found in patients with hypercalcemia.
a, b, and c. Hyperactive deep tendon reflexes, prolonged Q-T interval on EKG, and muscle weakness are commonly assessed in patients with hypocalcemia.
Analysis/Physiologic/Assessment

4. ***Correct response: a***
Canned fish is high in calcium.
b. Coffee is high in potassium
c. and d. Dry beans and meat are high in phosphorous.
Comprehension/Health Promotion/Implementation

5. ***Correct response: b***
IV calcium gluconate is used for replacement in severe cases of hypocalcemia.
a. Exercise, not bedrest would be rec-

ommended to release calcium from the bone into the serum.
c and d. Calcitonin and loop diuretics are used to lower serum calcium levels.
Application/Safe Care/Implementation

6. ***Correct response: c***
Lasix is a loop diuretic; this type of diuretic facilitates calcium removal.
a and b. These drugs will not facilitate calcium removal.
d. Mannitol is an osmotic diuretic, and treatment of hypercalcemia requires administration of a loop diuretic.
Application/Safe Care/Planning

7. ***Correct response: d***
Hypercalcemia causes cardiac dysrhythmias, reflected in a shortened Q-T interval.
a and b. Constipation and muscle weakness are sequelae of hypercalcemia, but are not dangerous.
c. Dyspnea is not a sequela of hypercalcemia.
Analysis/Physiologic/Analysis

8. ***Correct response: d***
Hyperparathyroidism accelerates parathyroid hormone (PTH) effects on bone and removes bound calcium into the serum.
a. Myxedema is associated with hypothyroidism. Hyperthyroidism, or thyrotoxicosis, is the direct opposite of hypothyroidism; it is thyrotoxicosis that places a patient at risk.
b. Exercise places a patient at less risk; immobility causes hypercalcemia.
c. Hypophosphatemia is associated with hypercalcemia.
Comprehension/Physiologic/Assessment

Magnesium: Normal and Altered Balance

9

I. Normal balance

A. Description

1. Magnesium is the second most abundant cation in the intracellular fluid.

2. Normal serum magnesium concentration ranges from 1.3 to 2.1 mEq/L.

B. Supply and sources

1. Magnesium is taken in through the diet and eliminated through the kidneys and gastrointestinal system.

2. Abnormal routes of magnesium intake include:
   a. IV administration
   b. Hyperalimentation

3. Sixty percent of total body magnesium is contained in bone.

4. Of all the serum magnesium, 33% is bound to protein; the remainder is ionized.

C. Functions

1. Exerts its effect on the myoneural junction, affecting neuromuscular irritability

Paradiso, C: *Lippincott's Review Series: Fluids and Electrolytes* © 1995 J. B. Lippincott Company

2. Assists in contraction of cardiac and skeletal muscle cells
3. Contributes to vasodilation and through this effect, changes blood pressure and cardiac output
4. Activates intracellular enzymes to participate in carbohydrate and protein metabolism
5. Facilitates sodium and potassium transport across the cell membrane
6. Influences intracellular calcium levels through its effect on parathyroid hormone secretion

  D. **Regulation**

1. Magnesium regulation is not clearly understood, but factors that influence the balance of other cations affect magnesium as well.
2. Magnesium levels are regulated by renal and extrarenal mechanisms:
   a. Magnesium is filtered along with all other electrolytes in the glomerulus.
   b. The amount filtered depends on the amount present.
   c. Magnesium is reabsorbed across all segments of the renal tubules.
   d. Tubular reabsorption is affected by the presence of the magnesium ion, especially in Henle's loop.
   e. When extracellular magnesium is high, excess magnesium is excreted.
   f. When extracellular magnesium is low, magnesium is conserved.
   g. Tubules can conserve magnesium so that daily losses can be reduced to 1.0 mEq/L per day.
   h. Diuretics that act on this region (eg, Lasix) can greatly increase magnesium excretion.

II. Magnesium deficiency: Hypomagnesemia

  A. Description: Serum magnesium levels less than 1.3 mEq/L

  B. Etiology

1. Magnesium loss, such as from:
   a. Severe GI fluid losses due to vomiting, diarrhea, gastric suctioning, or diuretics
   b. Ulcerative colitis
   c. Burns and débridement therapy
2. Inadequate intake or absorption due to:
   a. Malnutrition or starvation
   b. Malabsorption syndrome
   c. Excessive dietary intake of calcium or vitamin D
3. Fluid and electrolyte shifts due to:
   a. Administration of hyperalimentation solutions that are magnesium deficient
   b. Hypercalcemia

    c. Hypoparathyroidism

    d. Hypoaldosteronism (in which sodium is not absorbed and therefore magnesium is not absorbed)

    e. High-dose steroid use

    f. Diabetic ketoacidosis

    g. Gentamicin administration

    h. Sepsis

    i. Pancreatitis

    j. Alcoholism

    k. Pregnancy-induced hypertension

C. Assessment findings

  1. Clinical manifestations may include vomiting or diarrhea; however, these symptoms may be the cause of hypomagnesemia.

  2. Because magnesium is required for neuromuscular and cardiac muscle contraction and for vasodilation, any alteration will affect those muscle systems; symptoms may include:

    a. Dysrhythmias

    b. Hypotension

    c. Tetany

    d. Memory loss

    e. Seizures

    f. Confusion

    g. Tremors

    h. Hyperactive deep-tendon reflexes

    i. Positive Chvostek's and Trousseau's signs

  3. Laboratory results reveal:

    a. Serum magnesium level below 1.3 mEq/L

    b. Hypocalcemia

    c. Hypokalemia

  4. Another diagnostic cue is electrocardiogram (EKG) changes, which reveal prolonged PR and T intervals, wide QRS complexes, depressed ST segment, and inverted T waves.

D. Potential nursing diagnoses

  1. High Risk for Injury related to memory loss, seizures, confusion

  2. Decreased Cardiac Output related to electrolyte imbalances

E. Interventions

  1. Prevent hypomagnesemia or ensure early detection by identifying high-risk patients (eg, those with anorexia, nausea and vomiting, and diarrhea) and providing appropriate patient education.

  2. Aid in achieving treatment objective of elevating the magnesium level within the range of 1.5 to 2.5 mEq/L.

  3. Monitor patients with hypokalemia for impending hypomagnesemia.

  4. Monitor patients receiving total parenteral nutrition without magnesium added.

   5. Monitor a patient with hypomagnesemia who is on digoxin for signs of digitalis toxicity.
   6. Monitor cardiac status.
   7. Institute seizure precautions.
   8. Administer magnesium replacement slowly as ordered; rapid administration can cause cardiac arrest.
   9. Monitor urine output, which must be at least 100 mL every 4 hours for adequate renal excretion of magnesium to occur.
  10. Assess deep-tendon reflexes; if reflexes are absent, hold the dose, and notify the doctor.
  11. Infuse 10% magnesium at rate no more than 1.5 mL/min.
  12. Monitor potassium levels closely.
  13. Assess for stridor, because hypomagnesemia may cause airway obstruction.
  14. Assess for dysphagia.
  15. Monitor vital signs and cardiac rhythms.
  16. Instruct the patient on diuretics about the dangers of hypomagnesemia.
  17. Teach the patient about foods high in magnesium (eg, green vegetables, nuts, and fruit).

F. Evaluation
   1. Serum magnesium level returns to a range between 1.3 and 2.1 mEq/L.
   2. The patient remains free from injury.
   3. The patient's cardiac output is normal.

III. Magnesium excess: Hypermagnesemia

A. Description: Serum magnesium level above 2.1 mEq/L

B. Etiology
   1. Magnesium gain, such as from:
      a. Medications (eg, antacids)
      b. Hyperalimentation administration
      c. Hemodialysis using hard water dialysate
   2. Inadequate excretion due to:
      a. Reduced renal output
      b. Renal failure
   3. Fluid and electrolyte shifts due to:
      a. Hypoadrenalism (by the same mechanism affecting potassium)
      b. Diabetic ketoacidosis (as glucose brings cations across the cell)

C. Assessment findings
   1. Because magnesium is responsible for neuromuscular transmission, symptoms of hypermagnesemia are similar to those of hyperkalemia. Clinical manifestations may include:
      a. Cardiac arrhythmias
      b. Hypotension

      c. Bradycardia
      d. Hypoactive deep-tendon reflexes
      e. Warm systemic sensation
      f. Depressed respirations
      g. Depressed neuromuscular activity
  2. Laboratory tests reveal serum magnesium level above 2.1 mEq/L.
  3. EKG reveals changes in PR interval, QRS complex, and Q-T

D. **Potential nursing diagnoses**
  1. Decreased Cardiac Output related to altered magnesium
  2. Ineffective Breathing Pattern related to depressed respirations

E. **Interventions**
  1. Prevent hypermagnesemia or ensure early detection by identifying high-risk patients (eg, those taking antacids for any reason or receiving hyperalimentation) and providing appropriate patient education.
  2. Administer calcium gluconate as ordered to antagonize the cardiac effects of magnesium and temporarily relieve symptoms.
  3. Assess neuromuscular system for deficits.
  4. Monitor vital signs and cardiac rhythm.
  5. Check medications for magnesium, especially in patients with renal disorders.

F. **Evaluation**
  1. Serum magnesium level returns to normal range.
  2. The patient's cardiac output is normal.
  3. The patient's breathing patterns are normal.

Bibliography

Alspach, J. G. (1991). *Core curriculum for critical care nursing* (4th ed.). Philadelphia: W.B. Saunders.

Brunner, L. S., & Suddarth, D. S. (1992). *Textbook of medical-surgical nursing* (7th ed.). Philadelphia: J.B. Lippincott.

Guyton, A. (1991). *Textbook of medical physiology* (8th ed.). Philadelphia: W.B. Saunders.

McCance, K. L., & Huether, S. E. (1994). *Pathophysiology: The biologic basis for disease in adults and children* (2nd ed.). St. Louis: Mosby–Year Book.

Metheny, N. (1992). *Fluid and electrolyte balance: Nursing considerations* (2nd ed.). Philadelphia: J.B. Lippincott.

STUDY QUESTIONS

1. Normal serum magnesium concentrations range from:
   a. 0.5 to 1.5 mEq/L
   b. 1.3 to 2.1 mEq/L
   c. 10.0 to 12.0 mEq/L
   d. 3.5 to 5.0 mEq/L

2. When assessing a patient for hypomagnesemia, the nurse would *not* expect to find:
   a. hypoactive deep tendon reflexes
   b. hypotension
   c. cardiac dysrhythmia
   d. seizures

3. Which of the following groups of patients would the nurse closely monitor as being at high risk for hypomagnesemia?
   a. constipated patients
   b. anorexic patients
   c. obese patients
   d. patients with vitamin D deficiency

4. Nursing interventions for a patient with hypomagnesemia include:
   a. rapidly infusing 10% magnesium IV
   b. increasing diuretic therapy
   c. observing for signs of digitalis toxicity
   d. administering calcium gluconate

5. Which of the following foods selected by a patient with hypermagnesemia indicate the need for additional education?
   a. green vegetables, nuts, and fruit
   b. milk and cheese
   c. orange juice and bananas
   d. bacon and eggs

6. Which of the following findings would the nurse expect to assess in a patient with hypermagnesemia?
   a. serum level 1.2 mEq/L
   b. tachycardia
   c. warm systemic sensation
   d. hypertension

7. When assessing a patient for hypermagnesemia, the nurse is aware that a patient with which of the following conditions is at low risk?
   a. diabetic ketoacidosis
   b. chronic heartburn
   c. hypokalemia
   d. hypoadrenalism

8. Nursing interventions for a patient with hypermagnesemia include:
   a. administering 10% magnesium
   b. withholding diuretics
   c. limiting antacids
   d. administering digitalis

ANSWER KEY

1. *Correct response: b*
Normal serum magnesium concentration ranges from 1.3 to 2.1 mEq/L.
a, c, and d. These are not normal magnesium levels.
Knowledge/Physiologic/NA

2. *Correct response: a*
Hyperactive deep tendon reflexes are found in this disorder.
b, c, and d. Hypotension, cardiac dysrhythmia, and seizures are also symptoms of hypomagnesemia.
Application/Physiologic/Assessment

3. *Correct response: b*
Patients at high risk for hypomagnesemia include anorexics, and those with nausea, vomiting, and diarrhea.
a, c, and d. Vitamin deficiency, obesity, and constipation do not increase the risk of magnesium imbalance.
Comprehension/Safe Care/Assessment

4. *Correct response: c*
It is important to observe a patient with hypomagnesemia who is taking digitalis for signs of digitalis toxicity.
a. The nurse should infuse 10% magnesium slowly.
b. Increasing diuretic therapy can produce hypokalemia, which would worsen hypomagnesemia.
d. Calcium gluconate is given in hypermagnesemia.
Comprehension/Physiologic/Implementation

5. *Correct response: a*
Green vegetables, nuts, and fruits are good dietary sources of magnesium and

would be contraindicated for a patient with hypermagnesemia.
b, c, and d. These responses are incorrect.
Comprehension/Health Promotion/Evaluation

6. *Correct response: c*
A warm systemic sensation is a common symptom of hypermagnesemia.
a. Serum magnesium level of 1.2 mEq/L indicates hypomagnesemia.
b. Bradycardia, not tachycardia is observed in hypermagnesemia.
d. Hypotension, not hypertension occurs in hypermagnesemia.
Comprehension/Safe Care/Assessment

7. *Correct response: c*
Patients with hyperkalemia, not hypokalemia, are at increased risk to develop hypermagnesemia.
a, b, and d. Diabetic ketoacidosis, increased ingestion of antacids (due to chronic heartburn), and hypoadrenalism also increase a patient's risk for hypermagnesemia.
Comprehension/Health Promotion/Assessment

8. *Correct response: c*
Limiting antacids, which are high in magnesium, is indicated for the patient with hypermagnesemia.
a. 10% magnesium infusion is used to treat hypomagnesemia.
b. Withholding diuretics would not help, since diuretics may be part of the treatment.
d. Digitalis is not part of the treatment for hypermagnesemia.
Knowledge/Safe Care/Implementation

Phosphorus: Normal and Altered Balance

I. Normal balance

A. Description

1. Phosphorus is the major anion in the intracellular fluid (ICF); its concentration inside cells is approximately 100 mEq/L.

2. Normal serum phosphorus concentration ranges from 2.5 to 4.5 mg/dL.

B. Supply and sources

1. Normal sources of phosphorus intake include almost all foods; dairy products are especially rich in phosphorus.

2. Abnormal sources of potassium intake include intravenous administration and hyperalimentation.

3. Eighty percent of phosphorus exists in bone, where it is combined with calcium.

4. The remaining 20% is found in the ICF and extracellular fluid.

C. Functions

1. Acts as the critical component of the phosphate buffer system to aid renal regulation of acids and bases

2. Is necessary for the creation of energy through cellular metabolism, in which enzymatic action splits the compound adenosine triphosphate to produce phosphate and energy
3. Is an essential component of bones and teeth
4. Maintains cell membrane integrity by binding with lipids to create the phospholipid cell membrane layer
5. Is critical for the metabolism of protein, carbohydrates, and fats
6. Is essential to the function of red blood cells, muscles, and the neurologic system
7. Is a component of DNA and RNA

   D. Regulation
1. Phosphorus is filtered by the glomerulus.
2. When glomerular filtration increases, phosphorus reabsorption decreases; when glomerular filtration decreases, phosphorus reabsorption increases.
3. Phosphorus is reabsorbed in the proximal tubule along with sodium.
4. When parathyroid hormone (PTH) is present, tubular reabsorption is inhibited, increasing phosphorus excretion.
5. PTH is secreted is response to lowered serum calcium levels and is inhibited with higher serum calcium levels. This PTH secretion in response to calcium helps regulate phosphorus, because phosphorus is found in proportions inversely reciprocal to calcium.

II. Phosphorus deficiency: Hypophosphatemia

   A. Description: Serum phosphorus level below 2.5 mg/dL

   B. Etiology
1. Inadequate intake or absorption, such as that due to anorexia or malabsorption syndrome
2. Excessive losses from the gastrointestinal or genitourinary tract, such as from vomiting or diuretic use
3. Electrolyte shifts in which cations are exchanged (eg, hypokalemia, hypomagnesemia, metabolic acidosis, respiratory alkalosis, hyperaldosteronism)
4. Administration of high carbohydrate solutions without phosphorus
5. Secondary to diseases such as alcoholism or acute gout
6. Endocrine disorders (eg, hyperparathyroidism)

   C. Assessment findings
1. Symptoms include:
   a. Fatigue
   b. Muscle weakness
   c. Paresthesias
   d. Hemolytic anemia
   e. Nystagmus
   f. Rapid, shallow respirations

       g. Confusion
       h. Platelet dysfunction
    2. Laboratory tests reveal:
       a. Serum phosphorus levels below 2.5 mg/dL
       b. Hypercalcemia
       c. Rising creatinine phosphokinase levels (if serum phosphorus level remains low)

D. **Potential nursing diagnoses**

    1. Ineffective Breathing Pattern related to rapid, shallow respirations
    2. Fatigue related to anemia
    3. High Risk for Injury related to platelet dysfunction and confusion

E. **Interventions**

    1. Prevent hypophosphatemia, and ensure early detection by identifying high-risk patients (eg, those receiving excessive phosphate-binding medications, such as aluminum hydroxide [Amphojel] and aluminum carbonate [Basaljel], or those with hypercalcemia) and providing appropriate patient education.
    2. Assist in the treatment objective of returning the serum phosphorus level to a range between 2.5 to 4.5 mg/dL.
    3. Assess for signs of hypercalcemia, which occurs in the presence of hypophosphatemia.
    4. Increase dietary intake of phosphorus.
    5. Administer parenteral phosphorus as ordered if the depletion is severe.

F. **Evaluation**

    1. Serum phosphorus level returns to a range between 2.5 and 4.5 mg/dL.
    2. The patient remains free of injury.
    3. The patient's breathing pattern is normal.

III. Phosphorus excess: Hyperphosphatemia

A. **Description: Serum phosphorus level above 4.5 mg/dL**

B. **Etiology**

    1. Increased intestinal absorption due to excessive intake of vitamin D
    2. Ingestion of excessive quantities of milk
    3. Ingestion of certain phosphorus-containing medications (eg, laxatives)
    4. Administration of phosphorus-containing enemas (eg, Fleet's Phospho-soda)
    5. Renal insufficiency or failure
    6. Cellular destruction (eg, cancer chemotherapy, trauma, rhabdomyolysis), which causes release of phosphates into the serum
    7. Hypoparathyroidism, in which decreased PTH levels reduce calcium concentration, which in turn causes hyperphosphatemia
    8. Conditions that result in osteoporosis, because phosphorus is removed from bone and enters the serum

C. Assessment findings
1. Manifestations may include:
   a. Muscle spasms, pain, or weakness
   b. Positive Chvostek's or Trousseau's signs
2. Long-term effects are seen in the form of soft-tissue calcification (eg, joints, blood vessels, cornea), usually in patients with renal failure.
3. Laboratory tests show serum phosphorus level above 4.5 mg/dL and the presence of hypocalcemia.

D. Potential nursing diagnoses
1. Pain related to muscle spasms
2. High Risk for Decreased Cardiac Output related to hypocalcemia

E. Interventions
1. Prevent hyperphosphatemia, and ensure early detection by identifying high-risk patients (eg, those with hypocalcemia) and providing appropriate patient education.
2. Assist in the treatment objective of reducing serum phosphorus levels to a range between 2.5 and 4.5 mg/dL.
3. Administer phosphate binding medications (eg, aluminum hydroxide) as ordered.
4. Administer calcium supplements along with phosphate binders as ordered for a patient with renal-related hyperphosphatemia.
5. Prepare the patient for hemodialysis, which may remove excessive phosphorus.
6. Instruct the patient to avoid foods and medications that contain phosphorus.

F. Evaluation
1. Serum phosphorus level returns to a range between 2.5 and 4.5 mg/dL
2. The patient's cardiac output is normal.
3. The patient is free of pain.

Bibliography

Alspach, J. G. (1991). *Core curriculum for critical care nursing* (4th ed.). Philadelphia: W.B. Saunders.

Brunner, L. S., & Suddarth, D. S. (1992). *Textbook of medical-surgical nursing* (7th ed.). Philadelphia: J.B. Lippincott.

Guyton, A. (1991). *Textbook of medical physiology* (8th ed.). Philadelphia: W.B. Saunders.

McCance, K. L., & Huether, S. E. (1994). *Pathophysiology: The biologic basis for disease in adults and children* (2nd ed.). St. Louis: Mosby–Year Book.

Metheny, N. (1992). *Fluid and electrolyte balance: Nursing considerations* (2nd ed.). Philadelphia: J.B. Lippincott.

STUDY QUESTIONS

1. Phosphorus is primarily excreted via the:
   a. skin
   b. liver
   c. intestines
   d. kidneys

2. When providing patient teaching about phosphorus-rich foods, the nurse would *not* recommend:
   a. green, leafy vegetables
   b. soft drinks
   c. liver
   d. cheese

3. Normal serum phosphorus concentration ranges from:
   a. 1.0 to 2.5 mEq/dL
   b. 2.5 to 4.5 mEq/dL
   c. 3.0 to 6.0 mEq/dL
   d. 5.0 to 9.5 mEq/dL

4. Conditions that result in osteoporosis may cause hyperphosphatemia because:
   a. Phosphorus is removed from the bone.
   b. Phosphorus replaces calcium in the bone.
   c. The medications used to treat osteoporosis may cause it.
   d. As calcium levels increase, so do phosphorus levels.

5. Symptoms of hypophosphatemia include all of the following *except:*
   a. hemolytic anemia
   b. muscle weakness
   c. nystagmus
   d. positive Trousseau's sign

6. Phosphorus is necessary for:
   a. energy creation
   b. electrolyte diffusion
   c. normal urine function
   d. adequate cardiac contraction

7. Which one of the following endocrine hormones helps regulate phosphorus levels?
   a. antidiuretic hormone (ADH)
   b. adrenocorticotropic hormone (ACTH)
   c. parathyroid hormone (PTH)
   d. growth hormone (GH)

8. When caring for a patient with hyperphosphatemia, the nurse should be prepared to administer which of the following medications?
   a. Inderal
   b. Tagamet
   c. Dilantin
   d. Basaljel

ANSWER KEY

1. **Correct response: d**
   Phosphorus is excreted via the kidneys; renal failure can result in hyperphosphatemia.
   a, b, and c. These responses are incorrect.
   Knowledge/Physiologic/Assessment

2. **Correct response: a**
   Green, leafy vegetables are not rich in phosphorus.
   b, c, and d. Soft drinks, liver, and cheese are phosphorus-rich foods.
   Application/Health Promotion/Implementation

3. **Correct response: b**
   Normal serum phosphorus concentration ranges from 2.5 to 4.5 mEq/dl.
   a, c, and d. These values do not reflect normal levels.
   Knowledge/Physiologic/Assessment

4. **Correct response: a**
   As calcium is lost from the bone, so too will phosphorus be lost.
   b, c, and d. These responses are incorrect.
   Analysis/Physiologic/Assessment

5. **Correct response: d**
   Positive Trousseau's sign is found in hypocalcemia; this would occur with hyperphosphatemia, not hypophosphatemia.
   a, b, and c. Hemolytic anemia, muscle weakness, and nystagmus are symptoms of hypophosphatemia.
   Analysis/Physiologic/Assessment

6. **Correct response: a**
   Phosphorus is necessary for the creation of energy through cellular metabolism, where adenosine triphosphate (ATP) is enzymatically split to produce phosphate and energy.
   b. Phosphorus is required to maintain normal cell membrane integrity, but is not directly responsible for diffusion.
   c. Phosphorus levels do not affect urinary system functioning.
   d. Although phosphorus is an intracellular electrolyte, it does not affect cardiac contraction.
   Knowledge/Physiological/Analysis

7. **Correct response: c**
   Parathyroid hormone (PTH) regulates phosphorus levels by its response to calcium, which then affects phosphorus. When calcium levels decrease, PTH is secreted, moving calcium from bone to serum. The presence of PTH inhibits tubular reabsorption of phosphorus, allowing more phosphorus to be excreted.
   a, b, and d. These hormones do not influence phosphorus levels.
   Comprehension/Physiologic/Analysis

8. **Correct response: d**
   Basalgel is a phosphate-binding medication; its use allows dietary phosphorus to be bound in the gut and excreted.
   a, b, and c. These drugs do not affect phosphorus levels.
   Application/Safe Care/Planning

Acid–Base Balance

I. Overview of acids and bases

A. Description

1. *Acids* are substances that can release hydrogen ions.
2. *Bases* (alkalis) are substances that can accept hydrogen ions; bases include bicarbonate (HCO_3) ions.
3. Carbon dioxide (CO_2 is considered to be an acid or a base depending on its chemical association. When assessing acid–base balance, it is considered an acid because of its relationship with carbonic acid (H_2CO_3). Because carbonic acid cannot be measured, CO_2 measures are used.
4. To maintain the balance between acids and bases, dynamic processes continually adjust the concentration of hydrogen ions (H^+) and hydroxide ions (OH^-) within body fluids.
5. A measure of the ratio between acids and bases or the concentration of hydrogen ions within body fluids is pH.
6. Normal values for blood pH range within a narrow margin:
    a. Normal values for arterial blood range from 7.35 to 7.45.
    b. Extreme high and low pH values (such as 6.8 or 7.8) are incompatible with life.
7. An abnormal increase in hydrogen ions or decrease in bicarbonate ions results in *acidosis*; pH values drop below 7.35. An abnormal decrease in hydrogen ions or increase in bicarbonate ions results in *alkalosis*; pH values increase above 7.45. (See Chapter 12, Alterations in Acid–Base Balance, for more information.)

Paradiso, C: *Lippincott's Review Series: Fluids and Electrolytes* © 1995 J. B. Lippincott Company

8. *Buffers* are chemicals that maintain pH by ensuring a stable hydrogen ion concentration.

B. **Supply and sources**
   1. Acids and bases are found in:
      a. Extracellular fluid (ECF)
      b. Intracellular fluid (ICF)
      c. Body tissues
   2. Foods can produce acids and bases as a result of metabolism:
      a. Meats provide a dietary source of acids; meat is the main metabolic source of hydrogen ions.
      b. Fruits provide a dietary source of bases.
      c. Vegetables can provide acids and bases.
   3. Certain activities or conditions that are characterized by fat metabolism (eg, strenuous exercise and states of starvation) can produce acids.
   4. Catabolic processes also are known to release organic acids into the ECF.
   5. CO_2 is produced as an acid and a base by normal cellular metabolism.

C. **Role**
   1. Assist in maintaining a stable concentration of hydrogen ions in body fluids
   2. Maintain pH and thereby provide the necessary environment for bodily functions (eg, cellular metabolism and enzymatic processes) to occur
   3. Provide a neutral environment
   4. Compensate for specific imbalances

II. **Acid–base balance**
   A. **Description**
      1. Acids are constantly being produced through bodily functions and processes.
      2. Balancing acids and bases requires acids to be neutralized or excreted.
      3. CO_2, an acid, and HCO_3, a base, are crucial in maintaining acid–base balance.
      4. Normally, acid–base balance is maintained when the ratio of bicarbonate (HCO_3) to carbonic acid (H_2CO_3) is 20 to 1. (Note that carbonic acid is measured by carbon dioxide.)
   B. **Acid–base balance measurement**
      1. Arterial blood gas (ABG) values are used to measure acid–base balance (Table 11–1).
      2. ABG values show:
         a. The amount of oxygen (O_2), a gas, in the serum
         b. The amount of carbon dioxide (CO_2), a gas, in the serum
         c. The pH, or percentage of hydrogen ions in solution

TABLE 11–1
Arterial Blood Gases

TERM	NORMAL VALUE	DEFINITION—IMPLICATIONS
pH	7.35–7.45	Reflects H^+ concentration; acidity increases as H^+ concentration increses (pH value decreases as acidity increases) ▶ pH < 7.35 (acidosis) ▶ pH > 7.45 (alkalosis)
$PaCO_2$	35–45 mm Hg	Partial pressure of CO_2 in arterial blood ▶ When <35 mm Hg, hypocapnia is said to be present (respiratory alkalosis) ▶ When >45 mm Hg, hypercapnia is said to be present (respiratory acidosis)
PaO_2	80–100 mm Hg (decreases with age)	Partial pressure of O_2 in arterial blood ▶ Any reading above 80 mm Hg (on room air) is considered acceptable ▶ In adults younger than 60 yr (on room air) <80 mm Hg indicates mild hypoxemia <60 mm Hg indicates moderate hypoxemia <40 mm Hg indicates severe hypoxemia ▶ Somewhat lower levels are accepted as normal in aged persons because there is some loss of ventilatory function with advanced age
Standard HCO_3	22–26 mEq/L	HCO_3 concentration in plasma of blood that has been equilibrated at a $PaCO_2$ of 40 mm Hg, and with O_2 to fully saturate the hemoglobin
Base excess (BE)	−2–+2 mEq/L	Reflects metabolic (nonrespiratory) body disturbances, which may be primary or compensatory in nature Always negative in metabolic acidosis (deficit of alkali or excess of fixed acids) Always positive in metabolic alkalosis (excess of alkali or deficit of fixed acids Arrived at by multiplying the deviation of standard HCO_3 from normal by a factor of 1.2, which represents the buffer action of red blood cells

Metheny, N. M. (1992). Fluid and Electrolyte Balance (2nd ed.). Philadelphia: J.B. Lippincott.

    3. ABG analysis reveals:
       a. If the patient has enough O_2 to maintain perfusion
       b. If enough CO_2 is being eliminated
       c. The ratio of hydrogen to bicarbonate

III. Acid–base regulation
A. Chemical buffer system
    1. Chemical buffers are present in all body fluids (ICF and ECF), tissue, and bone.
    2. The chemical buffer system functions primarily to maintain a constant serum pH; to do this, buffers continually accept or release free hydrogen ions.

3. The three major buffer systems include:
  a. Carbonic acid–bicarbonate buffer system
  b. Phosphate buffer system
  c. Protein buffer system

4. The *carbonic acid–bicarbonate buffer system* is the primary ECF buffer. It is characterized by a series of chemical reactions between carbonic acid (H_2CO_3) and bicarbonate (HCO_3).

5. The *phosphate buffer system* buffers the ICF and ECF. A series of chemical reactions between buffering salts and hydrogen ions work to maintain pH.

6. The *protein buffer system* is a powerful and abundant ICF buffer. It works similarly to the carbonic acid–bicarbonate buffer system.

7. Bone buffers also can contribute to the buffering of acids and bases.

8. All of the chemical buffer systems work interdependently and require respiratory and renal regulation as well to maintain acid–base balance.

9. Table 11–2 provides more information about the chemical buffer system.

TABLE 11–2.
Chemical Buffer System

Carbonic Acid–Bicarbonate Buffer System	Handles more than 50% of all chemical buffer activities
	Takes place in body fluids and renal tubules
	Is illustrated by the following chemical expression: $CO_2 + H_2O \leftrightarrow H_2CO_3 \leftrightarrow H^+ + HCO_3^-$
	Involves Na, K, Ca, Cl, and Mg when changes in the chemical buffering system are underway, thereby affecting pH, acid–base balance, and electrolyte balance
Phosphate Buffer System	Takes place in body fluids and renal tubules
	Provides important buffering effects in the kidney's tubular fluid
	Results in pH adjustments through the reactions of dihydrogen phosphate ions and monohydrogen phosphate ions with acids or bases
	Is important in maintaining urine pH
Protein Buffer System	Performs the majority of ICF buffering
	Takes place inside the cells
	Works similarly to carbonic acid–bicarbonate buffer system
	Uses hemoglobin, which acts as an immediate protein buffer for volatile acids
Bone Buffer System	Takes place in bone and ECF
	Increases the use of bone carbonate when CRF is present; chronic buffering by bone is, in part, an etiology for various bone diseases occurring with CRF

Key: ICF, intracellular fluid; ECF, extracellular fluid; CRF, chronic renal failure

B. Respiratory regulation
1. The respiratory center in the medulla and the lungs is involved in respiratory regulation and compensation of the acid–base balance.
2. The lungs use carbon dioxide (CO_2) to regulate hydrogen ion concentration.
3. Through changes in the rate and depth of respirations, acid–base balance is achieved through CO_2 elimination or retention.
4. This respiratory regulation process occurs within minutes.
5. Changes in respiratory status for any reason can lead to changes in pH.
6. Compensation occurs in response to metabolic disturbances. It occurs within minutes but is only a temporary or limited response.

C. Renal regulation
1. Renal regulation of acid–base balance (Table 11–3) is achieved by three interrelated processes:
   a. Bicarbonate reabsorption
   b. Bicarbonate formation
   c. Hydrogen ion excretion
2. *Bicarbonate reabsorption* occurs in the proximal tubule; it requires secretion of hydrogen ions by the kidneys and the enzymatic action of carbonic anhydrase. The reabsorbed bicarbonate is returned to body fluids, where it is available for the chemical buffer system.
3. *Bicarbonate production* is needed to replace the bicarbonate that

TABLE 11–3.
Renal Regulation

Bicarbonate Reabsorption	Secreted hydrogen ions combine with bicarbonate to form carbonic acid. Carbonic anhydrase reacts with carbonic acid to form water and carbon dioxide. The water is excreted, and the carbon dioxide diffuses to the tubular cells. Carbonic anhydrase reacts with carbon dioxide to form bicarbonate, which can be reabsorbed by the proximal tubules and returned to body fluids.
Bicarbonate Production	Hydrogen ions are secreted. Carbonic acid dissociates into hydrogen ions and bicarbonate. Hydrogen ions are excreted. Bicarbonate moves to the peritubular capillary.
Hydrogen Ion Excretion	Ammonia (NH_3) combines with hydrogen ions to form ammonium (NH_4). NH_4 cannot cross cell membranes and is excreted. Similar excretion of hydrogen ions is achieved with phosphates and titratable acids.

has been used to maintain the bicarbonate concentration; this is done by the kidneys. Bicarbonate produced by the kidneys increases the plasma concentration.

4. The production of bicarbonate also involves secretion of hydrogen ions.

5. Hydrogen ions accumulate from dietary, metabolic, and secretory sources.

6. *Hydrogen ion excretion* helps maintain acid–base balance. When excessive amounts of hydrogen are present, the volume delivered to the kidneys is high, creating an acidic glomerular filtrate and subsequently acidic urine.

7. Hydrogen ions also are excreted after they are buffered with ammonia.

8. Compensation for metabolic disturbances in acid–base balance is provided by the kidneys.

Bibliography

Brunner, L. S., & Suddarth, D. S. (1988). *Textbook of medical-surgical nursing* (6th ed.). Philadelphia: J.B. Lippincott.

Fischbach, F. (1988). *A manual of laboratory diagnostic tests* (3rd ed.). Philadelphia: J.B. Lippincott.

Holmes, O. (1993). *Human acid-base physiology: A student text.* London: Chapman & Hall Medical.

Horne, M. M., Heitz, U. E., & Swearingen, P. L. (1991). *Fluid, electrolyte, and acid-base balance: A case study approach.* St. Louis: Mosby–Year Book.

Lowenstein, J. (1993). *Acid and basics: A guide to understanding acid-base disorders.* New York: Oxford University Press.

STUDY QUESTIONS

1. Which of the following systems is *not* involved in maintaining acid–base balance?
   a. respiratory
   b. chemical
   c. blood
   d. renal

2. Normal values for arterial blood pH range from:
   a. 7.31 to 7.41
   b. 7.35 to 7.45
   c. 6.8 to 7.8
   d. 7.5 to 8.0

3. Balancing acids and bases requires neutralization or excretion of acids because:
   a. Acids are stronger than bases.
   b. The body is constantly producing acids through body functions and processes.
   c. All foods produce acids.
   d. Acids are toxic to body tissues.

4. Chemical buffers function to:
   a. Maintain a constant serum pH.
   b. Accept or release free hydroxide ions.
   c. Remain dormant until needed to re-balance acid and bases.
   d. Eliminate or retain CO_2 to maintain balance.

5. When assessing acid–base balance, the nurse would consider which of the following to be an acid?
   a. carbon dioxide
   b. sodium bicarbonate
   c. oxygen
   d. calcium phosphate

6. A nurse caring for a patient who is in a state of excessive catabolism (accelerated breakdown of proteins) knows that this patient may be at risk for:
   a. alkalosis
   b. acidosis
   c. hypoxia
   d. hypercapnia

7. Which of the following conditions may produce acids?
   a. resting
   b. overeating
   c. starvation
   d. obesity

8. Which is the primary extracellular fluid (ECF) buffer system?
   a. phosphate buffer system
   b. carbonic acid buffer system
   c. protein buffer system
   d. ammonia buffer system

ANSWER KEY

1. **Correct response: c**
   Blood is not one of the regulation systems involved in maintaining acid–base balance.
   a, b, and d. The respiratory, chemical, and renal systems are involved in maintaining the body's acid–base balance.
   Comprehension/Physiologic/Analysis

2. **Correct response: b**
   Normal arterial pH, a measure of the ratio between acids and bases, ranges from 7.35 to 7.45.
   a, c, and d. These are incorrect.
   Knowledge/Physiologic/Assessment

3. **Correct response: b**
   The body is constantly producing acids through body functions and processes. Balancing acids and bases requires neutralization or excretion of acids.
   a, c, and d. These are incorrect.
   Analysis/Physiologic/Analysis

4. **Correct response: a**
   Chemical buffers function to accept or release free hydrogen ions in an attempt to maintain acid–base balance and a normal pH.
   b. Chemical buffers accept or release hydrogen ions, not hydroxide ions.
   c. Chemical buffers are constantly in action.
   d. This response is incorrect.
   Comprehension/Physiologic/Analysis

5. **Correct response: a**
   When assessing acid–base balance, carbon dioxide is considered to be an acid because of its relationship with carbonic acid (H_2CO_3).
   b and d. These are not considered in the arterial blood gas (ABG) assessment.
   c. This response is incorrect.
   Knowledge/Physiologic/Assessment

6. **Correct response: b**
   Catabolic processes are known to release organic acids into the ECF.
   a, c, and d. These conditions may be revealed by ABG assessment, but are not related to catabolism.
   Comprehension/Safe Care/Analysis

7. **Correct response: c**
   Starvation causes fat metabolism, which results in the liberation of acids.
   a, b, and d. Resting, overeating, and obesity have no effect on acid production.
   Knowledge/Physiologic/Analysis.

8. **Correct response: b**
   The carbonic acid-bicarbonate buffer system is the primary ECF buffer. It is characterized by a series of chemical reactions between carbonic acid and bicarbonate.
   a. Although the phosphate buffer system works in the ECF and ICF, it remains secondary to the carbonic acid–bicarbonate buffer system.
   c and d. These buffer systems are secondary to the carbonic acid–bicarbonate buffer system and work in the intracellular space.
   Knowledge/Physiologic/Analysis

Alterations in Acid–Base Balance

I. Introduction

A. Overview

1. Acid–base balance is necessary to maintain homeostasis in the body's fluids.

2. Alterations in acid–base balance result in changes in certain bodily functions (eg, respiratory stimulation, maintenance of electrolyte balance).

3. *Acidosis* refers to an abnormal increase in hydrogen ions or decrease in bicarbonate ions.

4. *Alkalosis* refers to an abnormal decrease in hydrogen ions or increase in bicarbonate ions.

B. Types of acid–base imbalances

1. Single acid–base imbalances include:

a. Respiratory acidosis
b. Respiratory alkalosis
c. Metabolic acidosis
d. Metabolic alkalosis

2. Metabolic acidosis may be classified into two types:
   a. Nonanion gap acidosis
   b. Anion gap acidosis, which is uncommon (see Display 12–1 for more information)
3. Mixed acid–base disorders occur when two or more single acid–base imbalances are present, causing arterial blood gas (ABG) abnormalities:
   a. To determine whether these changed ABG values relate to compensation or represent the emergence of a second acid–base imbalance, the nurse must conduct a careful assessment. (Display 12–2 outlines the necessary steps in the ABG assessment.)
   b. Clinical conditions associated with mixed acid–base imbalances include cardiopulmonary distress, renal failure with gastric drainage and vomiting, renal failure with chronic obstructive pulmonary disease (COPD), COPD with vomiting, and renal failure with pneumonia. Any coexisting respiratory disorder can yield a mixed acid–base disorder.

II. Respiratory acidosis
A. Description
1. Respiratory acidosis is an acid–base imbalance caused by a decrease in pulmonary ventilation (eg, hypoventilation).
2. Hypoventilation increases carbon dioxide (CO_2) concentration in the lungs and blood.
3. Increased carbon dioxide concentration increases the level of carbonic acid (H_2CO_2) and hydrogen ions circulating in the blood, lowering arterial pH levels toward 7.0.

DISPLAY 12–1.
Anion Gap Metabolic Acidosis

▶ Anion gap refers to the difference between anions and cations in the ECF; it can be calculated as follows:
anion gap = Na – (Cl + HCO$_3$) = 12 ± 2 mEq/L
(The difference between anions and cations must equal 12 [plus or minus 2].)
▶ When an anion gap is greater than 12, the ratio of anions to cations is increased, setting homeostatic mechanisms off balance and resulting in acidosis. The higher the gap, the worse the acidosis.
▶ Conditions that cause anion gap acidosis include *diabetic ketoacidosis* (in which ketones are produced in large amounts), *lactic acidosis* (in which excess lactic acid is produced due to poor tissue perfusion), and *salicylate intoxication* (due to the highly acidic metabolites produced by salicylate breakdown).

DISPLAY 12–2.
Systematic Assessment of Arterial Blood Gases

The following steps are recommended to evaluate arterial blood gas values. They are based on the assumption that the average values are

$$pH = 7.4$$
$$PaCO_2 = 40 \text{ mm Hg}$$
$$HCO_3 = 24 \text{ mEq/L}$$

I. *First, look at the pH.* It can be high, low, or normal as follows:

$$pH > 7.4 \text{ (alkalosis)}$$
$$pH < 7.4 \text{ (acidosis)}$$
$$pH = 7.4 \text{ (normal)}$$

A normal pH may indicate perfectly normal blood gases, or it may be an indication of a *compensated* imbalance. A compensated imblance is one in which the body has been able to correct the pH by either respiratory or metabolic changes (depending on the primary problem). For example, a patient with primary metabolic acidosis starts out with a low bicarbonate level but a normal carbon dioxide level. Soon afterward, the lungs try to compensate for the imbalance by exhaling large amounts of carbon dioxide (hyperventilation). Another example, a patient with primary respiratory acidosis starts out with a high carbon dioxide level; soon afterward, the kidneys attempt to compensate by retaining bicarbonate. If the compensatory maneuver is able to restore the bicarbonate: carbonic acid ratio back to 20 : 1, full compensation (and thus normal pH) will be achieved.

II. *The next step is to determine the primary cause of the disturbance. This is done by evaluating the $PaCO_2$ and HCO_3 in relation to the pH.*
   pH > 7.4 (alkalosis)
   1. If the $PaCO_2$ is < 40 mm Hg, the primary disturbance is respiratory alkalosis. (This situation occurs when a patient hyperventilates and "blows off" too much carbon dioxide. Recall that carbon dioxide dissolved in water becomes carbonic acid, the acid side of the "carbonic acid : base bicarbonate" buffer system.)
   2. If the HCO_3 is > 24 mEq/L, the primary disturbance is metabolic alkalosis. (This situation occurs when the body gains too much bicarbonate, an alkaline substance. Bicarbonate is the basic, or alkaline side of the "carbonic acid–base : bicarbonate buffer system.")
   pH < 7.4 (acidosis)
   1. If the $PaCO_2$ is > 40 mmHg, the primary disturbance is respiratory acidosis. (This situation occurs when a patient hypoventilates and thus retains too much carbon dioxide, an acidic substance.)
   2. If the HCO_3 is < 24 mEq/L, the primary disturbance is metabolic acidosis. (This situation occurs when the body's bicarbonate level drops, either because of direct bicarbonate loss or because of gains of acids such as lactic acid or ketones).

III. *The next step involves determining if compensation has begun.*
   This is done by looking at the value other than the primary disorder. If it is moving in the same direction as the primary value, compensation is underway. Consider the following gases:
   Example:

pH	PaCO$_2$	HCO$_3$
(1) 7.20	60 mm Hg	24 mEq/L
(2) 7.40	60 mm Hg	37 mEq/L

The first set (1) indicates acute respiratory acidosis without compensation (the $PaCO_2$ is high, the HcO_3 is normal). The second set (2) indicates chronic respiratory acidosis. Note that compensation has taken place; that is, the HCO_3 has elevated to an appropriate level to balance the high $PaCO_2$ and produce a normal pH.

Metheny, N. M. (1992). Fluid and Electrolyte Balance (2nd ed.). Philadelphia: J.B. Lippincott.

4. The body tries to restore normal pH by a process called compensation, which occurs in the kidneys:
   a. Compensation is achieved by reducing the amount of bicarbonate (HCO_3) ions excreted in the kidney.
   b. This occurs through increased renal absorption of bicarbonate.

B. Etiology

1. Any factor that interferes with the exchange of gases between blood and air present in alveolus can result in respiratory acidosis. These causes can be acute or chronic, but all are related to a state of hypoventilation.
2. Acute causes include:
   a. Cardiopulmonary arrest
   b. Pneumothorax or hydrothorax
   c. Chest wall trauma
   d. Acute abdominal distention
   e. Drug overdose (eg, sedatives, anesthesia)
   f. Airway obstruction
   g. Pulmonary edema
   h. Atelectasis
   i. Pneumonia
   j. Acute neurologic dysfunction from any cause (eg, cerebral trauma, Guillain-Barré syndrome).
3. Chronic causes include:
   a. Chronic emphysema and bronchitis
   b. Myasthenia gravis
   c. Cystic fibrosis
   d. COPD
   e. Congestive heart failure
   f. Pulmonary fibrosis

C. Assessment findings

1. Symptoms result as acids accumulate and serum pH decreases; as the pH level drops, symptoms progress in severity.
2. Symptoms can include:
   a. Tachycardia
   b. Dyspnea
   c. Slow, shallow respirations
   d. Tremors
   e. Confusion
   f. Dizziness
   g. Asterixis
   h. Altered level of consciousness
   i. Convulsions
   j. Warm, flushed skin
   k. Cyanosis

3. Laboratory findings in respiratory acidosis reveal alterations in normal ABG values for pH and $PaCO_2$ (Table 12–1):
   a. The pH is below 7.35; the lower the pH, the more severe the acidosis.
   b. $PaCO_2$ is above 42, indicating acids (CO_2) are being retained and that this is the cause of decreased pH.
   c. HCO_3 is normal, indicating that there is no metabolic component.
4. As renal compensation occurs, the pH moves closer to normal. Increasing levels of bicarbonate (due to renal absorption of bicarbonate) move the pH in a normal direction.
5. ABG results reveal the level of compensation at the time the specimen is taken; a normal pH indicates full compensation.

TABLE 12–1.
Acid–Base Imbalances: Arterial Blood Gas Analysis

DISORDER	pH	$PaCO_2$	HCO_3
Respiratory acidosis (uncompensated)	Below 7.35	Above 42	Normal
Respiratory acidosis (partially uncompensated)	Below 7.35	Above 42	Above 26 (Bicarbonate is retained to buffer the acid [CO_2] and move the pH to normal.)
Respiratory acidosis (fully compensated)	Normal	Above 42	Above 26
Respiratory alkalosis (uncompensated)	Above 7.45	Below 38	Normal
Respiratory alkalosis (partially compensated)	Above 7.45	Below 38	Below 22 (The kidneys eliminate bicarbonate to balance with the lowered acid levels, moving the pH toward normal.)
Respiratory alkalosis (fully compensated)	Normal	Below 38	Below 22
Metabolic acidosis (uncompensated)	Below 7.35	Normal	Below 22
Metabolic acidosis (partially compensated)	Below 7.35	Below 38	Below 22 (The respiratory system responds by hyperventilating, which eliminates the acid CO_2 in an attempt to eliminate extra acids and move the pH toward normal.)
Metabolic acidosis (fully compensated)	Normal	Below 38	Below 22
Metabolic alkalosis (uncompensated)	Above 7.45	Normal	Above 26
Metabolic alkalosis (partially compensated)	Above 7.45	Above 42	Above 26 (The respiratory system responds by hypoventilating to retain more acid so that the extra bicarbonate will be buffered, moving the pH toward normal.)
Metabolic alkalosis (fully compensated	Normal	Above 42	Above 26

D. Potential nursing diagnoses
1. Activity Intolerance
2. Ineffective Breathing Pattern
3. Altered Tissue Perfusion

E. Interventions
1. Plan the patient's activities to allow for rest intervals.
2. Keep needed objects within the patient's easy reach.
3. Position the patient in semi-Fowler's position to ease the work of breathing.
4. Encourage deep breathing, coughing, and changes in position at least every 2 hours.
5. Institute chest physiotherapy.
6. Suction airway to maintain patency.
7. Provide emotional support and reassurance to allay anxiety.
8. Monitor respiratory rate and depth frequently depending on each case.
9. Administer low flow oxygen therapy as ordered.
10. Monitor ABG levels for changes in pH and CO_2.
11. Force fluids (2 to 3 L daily, unless contraindicated) to loosen secretions and aid in expectoration.

F. Evaluation
1. Normal exchange of oxygen and carbon dioxide occurs.
2. The patient achieves maximum ventilation.
3. The patient reports no dyspnea.
4. ABG values return to normal ranges.

III. Respiratory alkalosis

A. Description
1. Respiratory alkalosis is an acid–base imbalance caused by an increase in the pulmonary ventilation rate (eg, hyperventilation).
2. Hyperventilation decreases serum carbon dioxide in the lungs and blood as carbon dioxide is eliminated with the excess respirations. (The ratio of CO_2 to bicarbonate then changes, with bicarbonate being excessive due to a loss of CO_2)
3. Decreased carbon dioxide concentration decreases the level of carbonic acid (H_2CO_3) and hydrogen ions circulating in the blood, raising arterial pH levels.
4. The body tries to restore the pH to normal through renal compensation; in this process, renal excretion of bicarbonate is increased.

B. Etiology
1. Any factor that contributes to hyperventilation, which lowers $PaCO_2$, can cause respiratory alkalosis.
2. Potential causes include:
   a. Acute hypoxia (eg, due to pneumonia, asthma, pulmonary edema)

      b. Chronic hypoxia (eg, due to pulmonary fibrosis, cyanotic heart disease, high altitudes)

      c. Anxiety

      d. Fever

      e. Aspirin overdose

      f. Central nervous system trauma or seizures

      g. Exercise

      h. Gram-negative sepsis

      i. Hepatic cirrhosis

      j. Excessive mechanical ventilation

      k. Pregnancy

C. **Assessment findings**

    1. Symptoms result as acids are reduced and bicarbonate accumulates; symptoms may include:

      a. Paresthesia

      b. Numbness and tingling

      c. Light-headedness

      d. Confusion

      e. Tetany and loss of consciousness (if alkalosis is severe)

    2. Laboratory findings reveal alterations in normal ABG values for pH and $PaCO_2$ (see Table 12–1):

      a. The pH is above 7.45; the higher the pH, the worse the alkalosis.

      b. $PaCO_2$ is below 38, indicating a loss of the acid CO_2.

      c. HCO_3 is normal, making the ratio of acids to bases excessive on the base side; a normal bicarbonate indicates that there is no metabolic compensation.

    3. As renal compensation occurs, the pH moves closer to normal as bicarbonate is excreted by the kidneys. A normal pH indicates full compensation.

D. **Potential nursing diagnoses**

    1. Ineffective Breathing Pattern

    2. High Risk for Injury

E. **Interventions**

    1. Assist in achieving the goal of reducing the ventilation rate or maintaining the balance.

    2. Encourage slow, deep breathing (use a paper bag or rebreathing mask, if necessary).

    3. Monitor vital signs, especially respiratory rate and depth.

    4. If sedation is used to slow respiratory rate, assess the patient for respiratory depression.

    5. Provide emotional support and reassurance to the patient to reduce anxiety.

    6. Institute and maintain seizure precautions.

    7. Assist the patient with activities of daily living.

F. Evaluation

1. The patient remains free from injury.
2. The patient displays regular respiratory rate and breathing pattern.
3. ABG values return to normal ranges.

IV. Metabolic acidosis

A. Description

1. Metabolic acidosis is an acid–base imbalance caused by an increased accumulation of metabolic acids (eg, lactic acid and ketoacids) that rise in proportion to bicarbonate, resulting in decreased arterial pH.
2. Electrolytes always compete with each other for binding. In instances of metabolic acidosis, chloride and bicarbonate compete to bind with sodium. Acidosis also allows more chloride to be present, accounting for increased acids.
3. A loss of bicarbonate ions (bases) also will cause acidosis because the acid–base balance is offset by the greater amount of acids present.
4. As the pH decreases with rising levels of acids (as compared with bicarbonate), the excess hydrogen ions stimulate chemoreceptors.
5. The chemoreceptors in turn increase the respiratory rate (hyperventilation), causing respiratory compensation. This occurs immediately at the onset of acidosis.
6. Hyperventilation occurs to compensate and lower the CO_2 levels, moving the ratio of CO_2 to H_2CO_3 toward normal.
7. After several hours of respiratory compensation, the pH returns to a range between 7.35 and 7.45.
8. Even though the respiratory system compensates, the underlying metabolic disturbance may still remain.

B. Etiology

1. Metabolic acid build-up occurs when:
   a. Metabolic demands are greater than carbohydrate stores or when carbohydrates are not used normally by body cells, resulting in fat metabolism (eg, ketoacidosis or starvation).
   b. Metabolism occurs anaerobically (lactic acidosis).
   c. The kidneys are unable to retain bicarbonate (eg, renal failure).
2. Other causes of metabolic acidosis include:
   a. Salicylate toxicity
   b. Loss of bicarbonate through the renal system (diuretics) or gastrointestinal system (diarrhea)
   c. Trauma or burns in which lactic acid is produced (due to lack of oxygen availability to the cells)

C. Assessment findings

1. Symptoms result as acids accumulate, changing the levels of other electrolytes, and as compensation occurs; symptoms may include:

    a. Kussmaul's respirations
    b. Fruity breath (when diabetic ketoacidosis is the cause)
    c. Lethargy
    d. Drowsiness
    e. Confusion
    f. Headache
    g. Stupor
    h. Seizures
    i. Twitching
    j. Nausea
    k. Vomiting
    l. Peripheral vasodilation
    m. Flushed skin
    n. Warm, dry skin
    o. Hyperkalemia or hyperchloremia (possible)

  2. Laboratory results reveal alterations in normal ABG values for pH and HCO_3 (see Table 12–1):
    a. The pH is below 7.35; the lower the pH, the more severe the acidosis.
    b. $PaCO_2$ is normal.
    c. HCO_3 is lowered.

  3. A normal $PaCO_2$ indicates that respiratory compensation has not occurred.

  4. Compensation occurs as the respiratory system increases its ventilation rate to blow off more acids (CO_2) in an attempt to eliminate excess acid and move the pH toward normal.

  5. A normal pH indicates full compensation.

D. **Potential nursing diagnoses**
  1. High Risk for Injury
  2. Altered Tissue Perfusion

E. **Interventions**
  1. Institute and maintain safety precautions (eg, side rails, seizure precautions).
  2. Monitor hemodynamic status through blood pressure and pulse rate and rhythm.
  3. Assess peripheral vascular status (eg, capillary refill, temperature, color).
  4. Monitor cardiac status.

F. **Evaluation**
  1. ABG values return to normal.
  2. Heart rate, rhythm, and blood pressure return to normal.
  3. The patient remains injury free.

V. Metabolic alkalosis

A. **Description**
  1. Metabolic alkalosis is an acid–base imbalance caused by an increased loss of acid (most often from the stomach or kidneys).

2. Loss of a fixed acid decreases the hydrogen ion concentration.
3. As the hydrogen ion concentration decreases, more carbonic acid breaks down, and serum bicarbonate concentration increases (because there is more concentration available, the kidney reabsorbs more). This results in increased excretion of the cations hydrogen, potassium, and chloride.
4. Because chloride and bicarbonate compete with each other for sodium binding, as chloride levels drop through binding, bicarbonate levels rise in compensation to balance the sodium.
5. As a result, chemoreceptor stimulation is decreased, lowering the respiratory rate.
6. Hypoventilation, the respiratory compensatory mechanism, keeps more acids in the body to balance the excess bicarbonate.
7. This occurs as hypoventilation reduces the amount of CO_2 that is eliminated, allowing more CO_2 (an acid) to be reabsorbed.

B. Etiology
1. Vomiting or gastric drainage
2. Diuretic therapy
3. Posthypercapnia alkalosis
4. Cushing's syndrome
5. Primary aldosteronism
6. Bartter's syndrome
7. Severe potassium depletion

C. Assessment findings
1. Symptoms may include:
   a. Apathy
   b. Confusion
   c. Stupor
   d. Tetany (if serum calcium is borderline low)
   e. Decreased respiratory rate and depth (may be a compensatory mechanism to conserve CO_2)
   f. Dizziness
   g. Paresthesia (in fingers and toes)
   h. Carpopedal spasm
   i. Nausea and vomiting
   j. Seizures
   k. Low serum potassium and chloride levels (related to sodium levels)
   l. Electrocardiogram changes (alterations in T and U waves may occur due to hypokalemia)
   m. Urine pH less than 7.0 (occurs in patients with sustained metabolic alkalosis because the serum delivered to the tubules is rich in bicarbonate, resulting in bicarbonate secretion)
2. Laboratory test results reveal alterations in normal ABG values for pH and HCO_3 (see Table 12–1):

      a. The pH is above 7.45; the higher the pH, the worse the alkalosis.

      b. PCO_2 is normal.

      c. HCO_3 levels are higher, indicating that the cause is metabolic.

  3. As respiratory compensation occurs, the PCO_2 levels rise to buffer the higher-than-normal HCO_3. A normal pH indicates full compensation.

D. **Potential nursing diagnoses**

  1. Ineffective Breathing Patterns

  2. High Risk for Injury

E. **Interventions**

  1. Monitor respiratory rate and pattern.

  2. Auscultate lung sounds.

  3. Ensure adequate hydration.

  4. Monitor intake and output.

  5. Monitor serum electrolytes.

F. **Evaluation**

  1. ABG and electrolyte values return to normal ranges.

  2. The patient's breathing patterns are normal.

  3. The patient is free from injury.

Bibliography

Alspach, J. G. (1991). *Core curriculum for critical care nursing* (4th ed.). Philadelphia: W.B. Saunders.

Brunner, L. S., & Suddarth, D. S. (1992). *Textbook of medical-surgical nursing* (7th ed.). Philadelphia: J.B. Lippincott.

Guyton, A. (1991). *Textbook of medical physiology* (8th ed.). Philadelphia: W.B. Saunders.

McCance, K. L., & Huether, S. E. (1994). *Pathophysiology: The biologic basis for disease in adults and children* (2nd ed.). St. Louis: Mosby–Year Book.

Metheny, N. (1992). *Fluid and electrolyte balance: Nursing considerations* (2nd ed.). Philadelphia: J.B. Lippincott.

STUDY QUESTIONS

1. A patient's arterial blood gas (ABG) values are pH 7.34, $PaCO_2$ 44, HCO_3 28; the nurse would analyze these findings as indicating:
   a. respiratory acidosis, uncompensated
   b. respiratory acidosis, partially compensated
   c. metabolic acidosis, uncompensated
   d. metabolic acidosis, partially compensated

2. When assessing a patient for respiratory alkalosis, the nurse would *not* expect to observe:
   a. paresthesias
   b. hypoventilation
   c. carpopedal spasm
   d. syncope

3. Nursing interventions for respiratory alkalosis include:
   a. cupping and clapping
   b. suctioning
   c. using a rebreathing mask
   d. administering oxygen

4. The body's compensation for respiratory alkalosis involves:
   a. decreased excretion of bicarbonate
   b. increased excretion of bicarbonate
   c. increased excretion of hydrogen ions
   d. increased retention of bicarbonate

5. When assessing a patient for metabolic acidosis, the nurse would expect to assess:
   a. carpopedal spasm
   b. tetany
   c. hypokalemia
   d. Kussmaul's respirations

6. Which of the following series of ABG values indicates uncompensated metabolic acidosis?
   a. pH 7.32, $PaCO_2$ 43, HCO_3 26
   b. pH 7.32, $PaCO_2$ 43, HCO_3 28
   c. pH 7.32, $PaCO_2$ 32, HCO_3 20
   d. pH 7.32, $PaCO_2$ 38, HCO_3 20

7. The body attempts to compensate for metabolic acidosis by:
   a. increasing the respiratory rate
   b. decreasing the respiratory rate
   c. increasing urinary output
   d. decreasing urinary output

8. Concomitant electrolyte alterations commonly observed in metabolic alkalosis include:
   a. decreased serum potassium and chloride
   b. increased serum potassium and chloride
   c. decreased serum sodium
   d. increased serum potassium and sodium

9. In reviewing the laboratory data for a patient with suspected respiratory acidosis, the nurse is aware that which of the following ABG components would confirm that the problem is, indeed, respiratory and not metabolic?
   a. pH
   b. $PaCO_2$
   c. HCO_3
   d. none of the above

10. Nursing interventions for a patient in respiratory acidosis with a nursing diagnosis of activity intolerance would include:
    a. suctioning airway to maintain patency
    b. forcing fluids
    c. instituting chest physiotherapy
    d. planning the patient's activities to allow for rest

ANSWER KEY

1. *Correct response: b*
   These ABG values indicate respiratory acidosis, partially compensated.
   a. ABG values of pH 7.34, $PaCO_2$ 44, HCO_3 26 indicate respiratory acidosis, uncompensated.
   c. ABG values of pH 7.34, $PaCO_2$ 38, HCO_3 20 indicate metabolic acidosis, uncompensated.
   d. ABG values of pH 7.34, $PaCO_2$ 36, HCO_3 20 indicate metabolic acidosis, partially uncompensated.
   Analysis/Safe Care/Assessment

2. *Correct response: b*
   Hyperventilation, not hypoventilation, is seen in respiratory alkalosis.
   a, c, and d. Paresthesias, carpopedal spasm, and syncope are observed in respiratory alkalosis.
   Application/Safe Care/Assessment

3. *Correct response: c*
   Use of a rebreathing mask allows the patient to increase his $PaCO_2$.
   a, b, and d. Cupping and clapping, suctioning, and oxygen administration are appropriate interventions for respiratory acidosis.
   Application/Safe Care/Intervention

4. *Correct response: b*
   Respiratory alkalosis involves an excessive amount of base in relation to acid; the body attempts to compensate by increasing base (bicarbonate) excretion.
   a, c, and d. These responses are incorrect.
   Comprehension/Physiologic/Analysis

5. *Correct response: d*
   Kussmaul's respirations are a classic sign of metabolic acidosis.
   a, b, and c. Carpopedal spasm, tetany, and hypokalemia are symptoms of metabolic alkalosis.
   Knowledge/Safe Care/Assessment

6. *Correct response: d*
   ABG values of pH 7.32, $PaCO_2$ 38, HCO_3 20 indicate metabolic acidosis.
   a. These ABG values indicate respiratory acidosis, uncompensated.
   b. These ABG values indicate respiratory acidosis, partially compensated
   c. These ABG values indicate metabolic acidosis, partially compensated.
   Knowledge/Physiologic Integrity/Assessment

7. *Correct response: a*
   The body attempts to compensate for metabolic acidosis by increasing the respiratory rate and therefore "blowing off" acid (carbon dioxide).
   b, c, and d. These responses are incorrect.
   Comprehension/Physiologic/Assessment

8. *Correct response: a*
   Decreased serum potassium and serum chloride are found in metabolic alkalosis.
   b, c, and d. These electrolyte fluctuations are not associated with metabolic alkalosis.
   Application/Physiologic/Assessment

9. *Correct response: c*
   The HCO_3 is normal, indicating that there is no metabolic component.
   a and b. Although laboratory findings in respiratory acidosis reveal alterations in pH and $PaCO_2$, the HCO_3 indicates a metabolic component.
   d. This response is incorrect.
   Application/Physiologic/Assessment

10. *Correct response: d*
    This is the only nursing intervention specifically related to the diagnosis of activity intolerance.
    a, b, and c. These nursing interventions may be appropriate for some of the respiratory-related nursing diagnoses.
    Application/Safe care/Implementation

—

IV Fluid Replacement Therapy

I. Introduction

A. Overview of intravenous (IV) fluid replacement therapy

1. IV fluid replacement changes the composition of the serum by adding fluids and electrolytes.

2. Consequently, the nurse must administer IV fluid replacement *with caution* to avoid adverse reactions, which can include:
    a. Fluid volume excess (FVE)
    b. Fluid volume deficit (FVD)
    c. Fluid shifts
    d. Decreased or increased electrolyte levels

B. Indications

1. Replacement of abnormal fluid and electrolyte losses, such as may result from surgery, trauma, burns, or gastrointestinal (GI) bleeding

2. Maintenance of daily fluid and electrolyte needs (eg, in situations in which the patient is unable to take in or tolerate oral food and

fluids [due to GI disorders], or the patient's status is nothing by mouth)

3. Correction of fluid disorders
4. Correction of electrolyte disorders (in conjunction with other therapies)

II. Types of solutions

A. Isotonic

1. An isotonic solution has the same osmolar concentration, or tonicity, as the plasma.
2. This means that the proportion of particles to solution infused is the same as that of the serum; as a result, fluid does not shift across the compartments, and the volume of fluid infused distributes equally across the intracellular and extracellular spaces.
3. Isotonic solutions include:
   a. 0.9% sodium chloride (normal saline)
   b. Lactated Ringer's solution

B. Hypotonic

1. Hypotonic solutions contain a lower osmolar concentration than the serum.
2. This means that the solution infused is more dilute than the plasma, containing more water than particles.
3. When hypotonic solutions are infused, fluid shifts from the extracellular space to the intracellular space to maintain equilibrium.
4. This eventually leads to swelling or "water logging" of the cells, known as water intoxication. (See Chapter 5, Sodium: Normal and Altered Balance, for more information.)
5. As the swelling increases, the cells eventually rupture.
6. Hypotonic solutions include:
   a. 5% dextrose and water (D_5W)
   b. 0.45% sodium chloride (half saline)
   c. 0.33% sodium chloride

C. Hypertonic

1. Hypertonic solutions have a higher concentration of particles in solution compared with the plasma.
2. To balance the concentration of fluid and particles across fluid compartments, fluid shifts out of the intracellular space into the extracellular space, causing cellular shrinkage or dehydration.
3. This cellular dehydration causes disturbances in the way cells function.
4. In addition, the shift of fluid out of the cells causes the extracellular compartment to expand, which, if excessive, can lead to FVE.
5. Hypertonic solutions include:
   a. 3% sodium chloride
   b. Protein solutions

    c. Hyperalimentation solutions of 10%, 50%, and 70% dextrose (see Display 13–1)

  6. Table 13–1 describes common isotonic, hypotonic, and hypertonic solutions.

D. Colloids

  1. *Colloids* are fluids that contain solutes of a higher molecular weight (eg, protein); this is in contrast to *crystalloids*, which are electrolyte solutions (eg, D_5W, lactated Ringer's solution, 0.9% normal saline).

  2. Colloid solutions have significant osmotic activity and are hypertonic.

  3. The presence of colloids in the vascular space pulls fluids from the interstitial and intercellular spaces.

  4. This osmotic activity makes colloid solutions useful for:

    a. Mobilizing third-spaced fluids

    b. Correcting hypotension

    c. Expanding intravascular volume

    d. Replenishing protein depletion (such as occurs with liver and renal disease, starvation, GI disease, and multisystem organ failure)

  5. Colloids include:

    a. Salt pour albumin

    b. Plasmanate

    c. Dextran

    d. Hetastarch (Hespan)

  6. Salt pour albumin contains a highly concentrated solution of albumin in a small volume of fluid.

  7. Plasmanate contains albumin, globulins, and fibrinogen, in a higher fluid volume than salt pour albumin.

  8. Dextran is a highly concentrated glucose solution; it may interfere with blood coagulation.

  9. Hetastarch also interferes with blood coagulation.

DISPLAY 13–1.
Hyperalimentation

- Hyperalimentation, or total parenteral nutrition, involves the parenteral administration of a hypertonic solution (eg, dextrose 50% or 70%) that contains all of the necessary dietary requirements (eg, proteins, carbohydrates, minerals, vitamins).
- The high-glucose solution provides a high-calorie intake and spares protein; in a patient who cannot eat, protein wasting may occur because carbohydrates and fats are burned first.
- Hyperalimentation is administered through a central venous catheter.
- Metabolic complications of hyperalimentation include hyperglycemia or electrolyte disorders if appropriate amounts of elements are not contained in the solution.

TABLE 13–1.
Contents of Selected Water and Electrolyte Solutions With Comments About Their Use

SOLUTION	COMMENTS
5% dextrose in water (D$_5$W) No electrolytes 50 g of dextrose	Supplies approximately 170 cal/L and free water to aid in renal excretion of solutes Should not be used in excessive volumes in patients with increased ADH activity or to replace fluids in hypovolemic patients
0.9% NaCl (isotonic saline) Na$^+$ 154 mEq/L Cl$^-$ 154 mEq/L	Not desirable as a routine maintenance solution because it provides only Na$^+$ and Cl$^-$, which are provided in excessive amounts
0.45% NaCl (½-strength saline) Na$^+$ 77 mEq/L Cl$^-$ 77 mEq/L	A hypotonic solution that provides Na$^+$, Cl$^-$, and free water Na$^+$ and Cl$^-$ provided in fluid allows kidneys to select and retain needed amounts Free water desirable as aid to kidneys in elimination of solutes
0.33% NaCl (⅓-strength saline) Na$^+$ 56 mEq/L Cl$^-$ 56 mEq/L	A hypotonic solution that provides Na$^+$, Cl$^-$, and free water Often used to treat hypernatremia (because this solution contains a small amount of Na$^+$, it dilutes the plasma sodium while not allowing it to drop too rapidly.)
3% NaCl Na$^+$ 513 mEq/L Cl$^-$ 513 mEq/L	Grossly hypertonic solutions used only to treat severe hyponatremia See Table 4–5 for summary of important nursing considerations in administration
5% NaCl Na$^+$ 855 mEq/L Cl$^-$ 855 mEq/L	Dangerous solutions
Lactated Ringer's solution: Na$^+$ 130 mEq/L K$^+$ 4 mEq/L Ca^{++} 3 mEq/L Cl$^-$ 109 mEq/L Lactate (metabolized to bicarbonate) 28 mEq/L	A roughly isotonic solution that contains multiple electrolytes in approximately the same concentrations as found in plasma (Note that this solution is lacking in Mg and PO$_4$.) Used in the treatment of hypovolemia, burns, and fluid lost as bile or diarrhea Useful in treating mild metabolic acidosis

Other isotonic multiple electrolyte solutions
Plasma-Lyte 148 (Baxter)
Isolyte S (McGaw)
Normosol R (Abbott)
Na+ 140 mEq/L
K+ 5 mEq/L
Mg++ 3 mEq/L
Cl- 98 mEq/L
HCO3 50 mEq/L (or equivalent)

Isotonic solution that can be used to replace ECF loss
Because of relatively high bicarbonate content, can be used to correct mild acidosis

Hypotonic multiple electrolyte solutions
Plasma-Lyte 56 (Baxter)
Normosol M (Abbott)
Na+ 40 mEq/L
K+ 13 mEq/L
Mg++ 3 mEq/L
Cl- 40 mEq/L
HCO3 16 mEq/L (or equivalent)

Hypotonic solution that supplies free water as well as electrolytes

Sodium lactate solution, 1/6 M
Na+ 167 mEq/L
Cl- 167 mEq/L

A roughly isotonic solution used to correct severe metabolic acidosis (lactate is metabolized to bicarbonate in 1–2 hr by the liver)
Not used in patients with liver disease (lactate cannot be converted to bicarbonate in such individuals); also, not used in patients with oxygen lack (unable to adequately convert lactate to bicarbonate)

Sodium bicarbonate, 5%
Na+ 595 mEq/L
Cl- 595 mEq/L

A very hypertonic solution used to correct severe metabolic acidosis
Should be cautiously administered at a slow rate, under careful volume control
Should be administered only with extreme caution to salt-retaining patients (eg, those with cardiac, renal, or liver damage)

Ammonium chloride, 2.14%:

Acidifying solution used to correct severe metabolic alkalosis
Due to high ammonium content, must be administered cautiously to patients with compromised hepatic function

Metheny, N. M. (1992) Fluid and Electrolyte Balance (2nd ed.). Philadelphia: J.B. Lippincott.

10. All colloids must be used *with extreme caution* because they move fluid from intracellular and interstitial spaces into the intravascular space, risking congestive heart failure and pulmonary edema.

III. Replacement with blood products

A. Indications

1. Blood products are required when large volumes of blood or body fluids have been lost.
2. To evaluate a patient's need for blood transfusions, the nurse would assess:
   a. Hemoglobin
   b. Hematocrit
   c. Cardiac output
   d. Swan-Ganz readings (if available)
   e. Vital signs
   f. Urinary output
   g. Skin perfusion
3. Blood transfusions are done only when absolutely necessary, and all blood donors are tested for the presence of human immunodeficiency virus.

B. Types of blood products

1. Types of blood products commonly used for transfusions include packed red blood cells (PRBC), fresh frozen plasma (FFP), platelets, and cryoprecipitate (Table 13–2); whole blood is rarely used as a transfusion.
2. *PRBCs:*
   a. Include a large volume of red blood cells (150 mL) in 100 mL of plasma
   b. Elevate hemoglobin levels quickly because they are so concentrated

TABLE 13–2.
Comparison of Blood Products

BLOOD PRODUCT	CONSTITUENTS	VOLUME (mL PER UNIT)
Packed red blood cells	Red blood cells Plasma (100 mL)	250 mL
Fresh frozen plasma	Plasma without red blood cells Plasma proteins Clotting factors (fibrinogen, albumin, and globulins)	200–250 mL
Platelets	Platelets only	50 mL
Cryoprecipitate	Fibrinogen Clotting factor VIII and XIII	10–25 mL

    3. *FFP:*
        a. Contains plasma proteins and clotting factors in a total volume of 200 to 250 mL.
        b. Is indicated in patients with large fluid volume losses and in those with coagulation disorders (eg, patients with liver disorders)
        c. Expands the ECF because it is hypertonic

    4. *Platelets:*
        a. Are highly concentrated in 50 mL
        b. Are indicated when platelet levels drop below 10,000 mg/dL
        c. Are administered as a separate transfusion

    5. *Cryoprecipitate:*
        a. Includes clotting factors and fibrinogen in 10 to 25 mL
        b. Is indicated when clotting profiles are so high; the patient may bleed to death

IV. **Starting an infusion**

  A. **IV equipment**
      1. Alcohol swabs
      2. Tourniquet
      3. Angiocatheters
      4. IV solution
      5. IV tubing
      6. IV extension tubing
      7. Infusion pump (optional)

  B. **Site selection**
      1. To select an appropriate vein, the nurse must assess the veins of both arms.
      2. Veins that are thin, scarred, or in poor condition should be avoided because they will not be able to accommodate the hydrostatic pressure caused by an infusion.
      3. Other factors to consider when selecting a vein include:
         a. Patient comfort and mobility
         b. Existence of other medical conditions (eg, postmastectomy status or presence of arteriovenous fistulas and grafts); in these conditions, an infusion is contraindicated on the affected side.
         c. Viscosity and content of the solution and rate of flow; thicker (eg, colloids or blood products) or irritating solutions (eg, potasisum chloride) will require larger veins.
      4. Common sites for IV cannulation include the lower cephalic or basilic veins in the lower forearm and the superficial veins of the hand (Fig. 13–1).
      5. An IV should not be inserted in the joint (elbow or wrist).

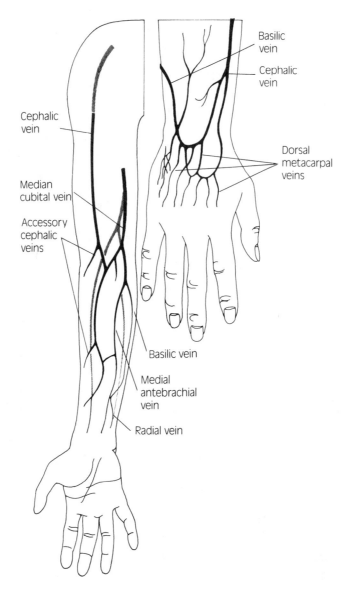

Basilic
vein

Cephalic
vein

Cephalic
vein

Dorsal
metacarpal
veins

Median
cubital vein

Accessory
cephalic
veins

Basilic vein

Medial
antebrachial
vein

Radial vein

FIGURE 13–1.
Infusion sites on the ventral and dorsal aspects of the lower arm and hand.

6. Central lines are specialized IV catheters that go into the central circulation:
   a. They may be inserted through the jugular or subclavian veins or through the periphery.
   b. The line passes into the vena cava just above the right atrium.

      c.   Because these types of catheters are more invasive, they are not appropriate for short-term use.

V. Nursing management

A. Initiating therapy

1. Ensure that the proper solution is prescribed to meet the patient's needs or that blood products have been properly typed and cross-matched.
2. Ensure that the catheter size is appropriate for the patient and for the vein selected.
3. Select a vein that is large enough to accommodate the fluid and that does not restrict mobility.
4. Maintain asepsis while preparing equipment, preparing the site, and inserting the catheter.
5. Take the patient's temperature before administering blood products.
6. Administer blood products with a filter so that no bacteria or small blood clots can pass through to the patient.
7. Be aware that different blood products infuse over different times:
   a. PRBC: Infuse over 2 to 4 hours
   b. FFP: Infuse over 1 to $1\frac{1}{2}$ hours
   c. Platelets: Infuse quickly
   d. Cryoprecipitate: Infuse quickly
8. See Display 13–2 for issues to consider when instituting IV therapy.

B. Monitoring therapy

1. Ensure that the IV catheter is secured.
2. Ensure that the appropriate solution or blood product is infusing at all times.

DISPLAY 13–2.
Intravenous Replacement Therapy: Questions to Consider

Before the Infusion:

► What is the patient's fluid status (eg, fluid volume excess or fluid volume deficit)?
► How much fluid can the patient's heart tolerate?
► How much fluid can the patient's kidneys tolerate?
► Does an electrolyte imbalance exist?
► Will the infusion cause a fluid shift?
► Is the solution or blood product appropriate for the patient's present condition?

During the infusion

► Does the solution or blood product being infused still meet the patient's current needs?

After the infusion:

► What effect has the infusion had on the patient?
► Has the treatment objective been achieved?

       3. Check that the flow rate remains appropriate.

       4. Monitor for signs of FVE or FVD.

       5. When blood products are used, take and record the patient's temperature during the infusion.

       6. Check hospital protocol to determine how often the dressing and catheter should be changed.

       7. Use aseptic technique when changing an IV dressing.

C. **Assessing for adverse reactions**

       1. Assess for FVE, which would occur if the patient's heart is unable to accommodate the amount of fluid given; symptoms can include:

          a. Full, bounding pulse

          b. Rales in the lungs

          c. Distended jugular veins

          d. Weight gain

       2. Assess for FVD, which would occur if too little fluid is given and the patient's fluid needs are not met; symptoms can include:

          a. Poor skin turgor

          b. Dry mucous membranes

          c. Tachycardia

          d. Hypotension

          e. Oliguria

D. **Handling complications**

       1. IV infusions:

          a. Local and systemic complications may occur as a result of IV therapy (Table 13–3).

          b. Common local complications include phlebitis and infiltration.

          c. Infection is a significant systemic complication that requires discontinuation of the infusion and immediate treatment of the pathogen.

       2. Blood transfusions:

          a. An increase in temperature indicates a possible transfusion reaction and requires immediate discontinuation of the infusion.

          b. Extreme transfusion reactions (eg, anaphylaxis) can be life-threatening (Table 13–4).

TABLE 13–3.
Complications Associated With Intravenous Infusions

NAME AND DEFINITION	CAUSES	SIGNS AND SYMPTOMS	NURSING CONSIDERATIONS
Infiltration: The escape of fluid into the subcutaneous tissue	▶ Dislodged needle ▶ Penetrated vessel wall	Swelling; pallor; coldness; or pain around the infusion site; significant decrease in the flow rate	▶ Check the infusion site often for symptoms. ▶ Discontinue the infusion if symptoms occur. ▶ Restart the infusion at a different site. ▶ Limit the movement of the extremity with the IV.
Phlebitis: An inflammation of a vein	▶ Mechanical trauma from needle or catheter ▶ Chemical trauma from solution ▶ Septic (due to contamination)	Local, acute tenderness; redness; warmth; and slight edema of the vein above the insertion site	▶ Discontinue the infusion immediately. ▶ Apply warm, moist compresses to the affected site. ▶ Avoid further use of the vein. ▶ Restart the infusion in another vein.
Thrombus: A blood clot	▶ Tissue trauma from needle or catheter shear	Symptoms similar to phlebitis IV fluid flow may cease if clot obstructs needle	▶ Stop the infusion immediately. ▶ Apply warm compresses as ordered by the physician. ▶ Restart the IV at another site. ▶ *Do not rub or massage the affected area.*
Fluid overload: The condition caused when too large a volume of fluid infuses into the circulatory system	▶ Too large a volume of fluid infused into circulation	Engorged neck veins; increased blood pressure; and difficulty in breathing (dyspnea)	▶ If symptoms develop, slow the rate of infusion. ▶ Notify the physician immediately. ▶ Monitor vital signs. ▶ Carefully monitor the rate of fluid flow. ▶ Check the rate frequently for accuracy.
Embolus: A foreign body or air in the circulatory system	▶ Thrombus dislodges and circulates in the blood ▶ Air enters the vein through the infusion line	Dependent on whether the embolism causes an obstruction or infarction in the circulatory system	▶ Check the site regularly to identify signs of phlebitis. ▶ Do not allow air to enter the infusion line. ▶ Treat phlebitis with the utmost caution. ▶ Report any sudden pain or breathing difficulty immediately.
Infection: An invasion of pathogenic organisms into the body	▶ Nonsterile technique used in starting infusion ▶ Improper care of infusion site ▶ Contaminated IV solution	Fever; malaise; and pain, swelling, inflammation, or discharge at IV insertion site	▶ Use scrupulous aseptic technique when starting an infusion. ▶ Change the dressing over the site regularly. ▶ Change IV tubing every 24 hours if agency policy permits. ▶ Always wash hands before working with the IV.

Taylor, C., Lillis, C. & LeMone, P. (1993). Fundamentals of Nursing (2nd ed.). Philadelphia: J.B. Lippincott.

TABLE 13–4.
Transfusion Reactions

REACTION	SIGNS AND SYMPTOMS	NURSING ACTIVITY
Allergic reaction: Allergy to transfused blood	Hives, itching Anaphylaxis	▶ Stop transfusion immediately and keep vein open with normal saline. ▶ Notify physician stat. ▶ Administer antihistamine parenterally as necessary.
Febrile reaction: Fever develops during infusion	Fever and chills Headache Malaise	▶ Stop transfusion immediately and keep vein open with normal saline. ▶ Notify physician. ▶ Treat symptoms.
Hemolytic transfusion reaction: Incompatibility of blood product	Immediate onset Facial flusing Fever, chills Headache Low back pain Shock	▶ Stop infusion immediately and kep vein open with normal saline. ▶ Notify physician stat. ▶ Obtain blood samples from site. ▶ Obtain first voided urine. ▶ Treat shock if present. ▶ Send unit, tubing, and filter to lab. ▶ Draw blood sample for serologic testing and send urine specimen to the lab.
Circulatory overload: Too much blood administered	Dyspnea Dry cough Pulmonary edema	▶ Slow or stop infusion. ▶ Monitor vital signs. ▶ Notify physician. ▶ Place in upright position with feet dependent.
Bacterial reaction: Bacteria present in blood	Fever Hypertension Dry, flushed skin Abdominal pain	▶ Stop infusion immediately. ▶ Obtain culture of client's blood and return blood bag to lab. ▶ Monitor vital signs. ▶ Notify physician. ▶ Administer antibiotics stat.

Taylor, C., Lillis, C. & LeMone, P. (1993). Fundamentals of Nursing (2nd ed.). Philadelphia: J.B. Lippincott.

Bibliography

Alspach, J. G. (1991). *Core curriculum for critical care nursing* (4th ed.). Philadelphia: W.B. Saunders.

Brunner, L. S., & Suddarth, D. S. (1992). *Textbook of medical-surgical nursing* (7th ed.). Philadelphia: J.B. Lippincott.

Guyton, A. (1991). *Textbook of medical physiology* (8th ed.). Philadelphia: W.B. Saunders.

McCance, K. L., & Huether, S. E. (1994). *Pathophysiology: The biologic basis for disease in adults and children* (2nd ed.). St. Louis: Mosby-Year Book.

Metheny, N. (1992). *Fluid and electrolyte balance: Nursing considerations* (2nd ed.). Philadelphia: J.B. Lippincott.

Taylor, C., Lillis, C., & LeMone, P. (1993). *Fundamentals of nursing: The art and science of nursing* (2nd ed.). Philadelphia: J.B. Lippincott.

STUDY QUESTIONS

1. Which of the following solution types is used to replace protein loss occurring secondary to liver disease?
   a. crystalloid
   b. colloids
   c. hypotonic
   d. isotonic

2. Cellular dehydration can result from infusion of:
   a. hypotonic solutions
   b. hypertonic solutions
   c. isotonic solutions
   d. plasmanate

3. Which of the following findings would the nurse *not* expect to assess in a patient with fluid volume excess (FVE)?
   a. rales
   b. bulging neck veins
   c. tachycardia
   d. weight gain

4. Nursing management for a patient receiving hypotonic fluids includes monitoring for which of the following potential complications?
   a. water intoxication
   b. FVE
   c. cellular shrinkage
   d. cell dehydration

5. The nurse would select which one of the following solutions for a patient who is to receive a hypertonic solution?
   a. 0.9% normal saline
   b. 5% dextrose and water
   c. 0.45% normal saline
   d. 3% normal saline

6. When administering a solution with the same osmolar concentration as plasma, the nurse is aware that:
   a. fluid will shift from the extracellular to the interstitial space.
   b. fluid will shift from the intracellular to the interstitial space.
   c. fluid will shift from the plasma to the intracellular space.
   d. no fluid will shift across compartments.

7. When selecting a site for intravenous fluid administration, the nurse would consider all of the following parameters *except:*
   a. body weight
   b. comfort
   c. prescribed infusion
   d. mobility

8. Which of the following solutions is a highly concentrated glucose solution that might interfere with coagulation?
   a. Plasmanate
   b. fibrinogen
   c. dextran
   d. salt pour albumin

9. A patient is receiving salt pour albumin every 4 hours. The nurse would monitor the patient for:
   a. renal failure
   b. diabetes
   c. congestive heart failure
   d. Cushing's syndrome

10. A patient will require an IV infusion of Plasmanate, and the nurse will start the infusion. The patient has a history of a right-sided mastectomy. The nurse should take which of the following actions?
   a. Start the IV in a large vein on the patient's left side.
   b. Inform the physician, since a central line will be needed.
   c. Start the IV in a smaller vein on the patient's right side.
   d. Start the IV with a small-gauge cannula on the patient's right side.

ANSWER KEY

1. *Correct response: b*
   Colloids are hypertonic solutions containing solutes of high molecular weight that pull fluids from the intracellular and interstitial spaces; these solutions are used to replenish protein depletion in liver and renal diseases.
   a. Crystalloids are intravenous solutions with solutes of lower molecular weight (e.g., 5% dextrose and water and 0.9% normal saline).
   c. and d. These are crystalloids.
   Application/Physiologic/Implementation

2. *Correct response: b*
   Hypertonic solutions produce a fluid shift out of the intracellular space into the extracellular space, causing cellular shrinkage or dehydration.
   a. Hypotonic solutions produce cellular swelling.
   c. Isotonic solutions produce no fluid shifts.
   d. This response is incorrect.
   Comprehension/Physiologic/Evaluation

3. *Correct response: c*
   Tachycardia and hypotension are seen in patient's with fluid volume deficit (FVD).
   a, b, and d. Rales, bulging neck veins, and weight gain are signs of FVE.
   Knowledge/Safe Care/Assessment

4. *Correct response: a*
   When hypotonic fluids are infused, fluid shifts from the extracellular to the intracellular space; eventually, this leads to swelling and water intoxication.
   a, c, and d. FVE, cellular shrinkage, and cell dehydration are potential complications of hypertonic fluid administration.
   Application/Safe Care/Evaluation

5. *Correct response: d*
   3% saline is a hypertonic solution; that is, it contains a higher concentration of particles in solution than plasma.

   a. 0.9% normal saline is isotonic.
   b and c. 5% dextrose and water and 0.45% normal saline are hypotonic.
   Application/Safe Care/Planning

6. *Correct response: d*
   Because isotonic solutions contain the same osmolar concentration or tonicity of plasma, administration of isotonic solutions results in no fluid shifting across compartments.
   a, b, and c. These responses are incorrect.
   Analysis/Safe Care/Evaluation

7. *Correct response: a*
   Body weight is not a usual consideration.
   b, c, and d. When selecting a site for IV infusion, the nurse should consider patient comfort, the prescribed solution (e.g., thicker solutions will require larger bore veins), and patient mobility (e.g., avoid a site over a joint).
   Knowledge/Physiologic/Assessment

8. *Correct response: c*
   Dextran is a highly concentrated glucose solution that may interfere with coagulation.
   a. Plasmanate contains albumin, globulins and fibrinogen.
   b. Fibrinogen is a component of plasmanate.
   d. Salt pour albumin contains a highly concentrated solution of albumin.
   Comprehension/Safe Care/Assessment

9. *Correct response: c*
   Salt pour albumin is a colloid, which is known to shift fluid from the intracellular and interstitial spaces into the intravascular space. This shift places the patient at risk for congestive heart failure or pulmonary edema.
   a, b, and d. These are not related to the risks of colloid use.
   Application/Safe care/Assessment

10. *Correct response: a*

The existence of other medical conditions is considered as part of IV site selection. A patient who has had a mastectomy should not have an infusion on the affected side.

b. There is no basis for this action.

c and d. Thicker or irritating solutions require larger veins.

Application/Safe care/Implementation

Assessing Fluid, Electrolyte, and Acid–Base Balance

Paradiso, C: *Lippincott's Review Series: Fluids and Electrolytes* © 1995 J. B. Lippincott Company

I. Introduction
A. Assessment goals
1. To assess a patient's potential or actual alterations in fluid, electrolyte, or acid–base balance, the nurse must conduct a thorough clinical assessment.
2. Specific assessment goals include:
   a. Ascertaining the body's capability to regulate fluid volume and body fluid composition
   b. Evaluating the body's effectiveness in maintaining normal acid–base balance
   c. Delineating specific aspects of fluid, electrolyte, or acid–base imbalance
   d. Identifying the severity of the fluid, electrolyte, or acid–base imbalance
   e. Determining the possible causes of abnormalities
   f. Incorporating appropriate nursing interventions into the patient's care plan

B. Assessment parameters
1. As suggested by Metheny (1992), the nurse must consider particular parameters when assessing a patient for fluid, electrolyte, and acid–base imbalances.
2. These key parameters include:
   a. Intake and output
   b. Urine volume and concentration
   c. Skin signs (eg, turgor, temperature, and moisture)
   d. Weight
   e. Subjective complaints of thirst
   f. Objective measures of fluid loss, such as tearing or salivation
   g. Edema
   h. Cardiovascular signs (eg, pulse, blood pressure, central venous pressure, and respirations)
   i. Neuromuscular signs

II. Intake and output
A. Normal findings
1. When measuring a patient's *intake*, the nurse should include:
   a. All fluids taken in by mouth or by intravenous, nasogastric, or nasointestinal administration
   b. Foods high in fluid content (eg, gelatin, ice cream)
   c. Electrolytes and nonelectrolytes ingested or administered
2. When measuring a patient's *output*, the nurse should include:
   a. Urine
   b. Fluid and electrolyte losses through the skin and gastrointestinal (GI) and respiratory tracts

      c.   Drainage from fistulas or body cavities

      d.   Fluids that have shifted into third spaces

  3. Because of the ability to concentrate fluids, normal kidneys maintain electrolyte and acid–base balance even when urine output is decreased to approximately 500 mL/d; as a person ages, urine-concentrating capability decreases.

  4. Normal intake should approximately match urinary output plus extrarenal losses.

B. **Altered findings**

  1. Decreased urine output and symptoms of dehydration

  2. Edema formation

  3. Altered amount of fluid and electrolyte excretion through the kidneys

  4. Oliguria or anuria

  5. Positive balance (occurs when intake exceeds output, including insensible loss)

  6. Negative balance (occurs when output exceeds intake)

C. **Possible causes of alterations**

  1. Excessive free water intake

  2. Inadequate intake

  3. Renal disease, such as:

      a.   Acute tubular necrosis

      b.   Acute renal failure

      c.   Chronic renal failure

      d.   Renal salt wasting

  4. Cardiovascular disease, such as:

      a.   Congestive heart failure (CHF)

      b.   Cardiomyopathy

  5. Iatrogenic administration of fluids

  6. Excessive nasogastric drainage

  7. Endocrine disorders (eg, syndrome of inappropriate antidiuretic hormone and diabetes insipidus)

  8. Frank blood or volume loss

  9. Third-space fluid shifting secondary to hepatic disease or due to fluid redistribution as found in burn injuries

  10. Causes of excessive extrarenal fluid losses can include:

      a.   Fever: Elevations in temperature result in increased fluid loss through the skin.

      b.   Hyperventilation: A ventilation rate that exceeds the body's metabolic needs results in increased insensible loss through the respiratory tract.

      c.   Ambient temperature: Hot, dry climates increase integumentary losses by evaporative processes.

      d.   GI losses: Diarrhea, vomiting, nasogastric drainage, and fistula drainage increase the amount of fluid and electrolyte losses.

e.   Distributive loss: Third-space shifting into pleural or peritoneal cavities, diffuse capillary leakage (as in liver or renal disease), and evaporative and transudative losses (as in a significant burn injury) increase fluid and electrolyte loss.

III.   Urine volume

A.   **Normal findings**

1.   In a patient with functioning kidneys, normal urine output is approximately 600 mL/d.

2.   Urine output will increase depending on the patient's intake and the amount of insensible loss.

3.   Baseline urine output in most clinical settings is approximately 30 mL/h.

B.   **Altered findings**

1.   Low urine volume

2.   High urine volume

C.   **Possible causes of alterations**

1.   Acute or chronic renal failure

2.   Fluid volume deficit (FVD) or fluid volume excess (FVE) due to any cause

3.   Redistributive conditions (eg, pancreatitis, burn injury, ascites, CHF)

4.   Diuresis

IV.   Urine concentration

A.   **Normal findings**

1.   The kidneys can reabsorb filtered water in relation to the degree of systemic hydration. The amount of fluid reabsorbed depends on the patient's hydration status and the amount of circulating ADH.

2.   The measure of urine concentration is the *specific gravity*. Specific gravity depends not only on hydration status, but also on the existence of solutes (eg, protein, glucose).

3.   A normal specific gravity is between 1.003 and 1.035.

4.   A more specific measure of concentration is *urine osmolality*, which is a measure of the total number of particles in solution, independent of the size and molecular weight of those particles.

5.   A normal urine osmolality depends on a number of clinical parameters, but an acceptable range is 50 mOsm/kg to 1200 mOsm/kg.

B.   **Altered findings**

1.   Elevated specific gravity and urine osmolality

2.   Low specific gravity and urine osmolality

C.   **Possible causes of alterations**

1.   Elevated findings may be associated with:

a.   Hypernatremia

  b. FVD
  c. Clearance of high–molecular-weight solutes (eg, contrast media)
2. Low findings may be associated with:
  a. Hyponatremia
  b. FVE
  c. Renal failure
  d. FVD

V. Skin turgor
A. Normal findings
1. Skin turgor indicates a patient's hydration status.
2. Skin with normal turgor moves easily when lifted and returns rapidly to its previous position.
3. Elderly patients tend to have less skin elasticity, so pinched skin returns more slowly to its normal position when released.
B. Altered findings
1. Poor skin turgor (eg, skin that remains elevated when lifted or "tents" or that takes a prolonged time to return to its normal position when released)
2. In edematous conditions, skin turgor that may be within normal limits but with fragile skin that is prone to breakdown
C. Possible causes of alterations
1. FVD
2. Peripheral edema

VI. Tongue turgor and mucous membrane moisture
A. Normal findings
1. Normally the tongue is covered with papillae on the dorsum and is smooth underneath.
2. In a patient with normal hydration, the tongue is moist and has no evidence of fissures (cracks in the surface).
3. The oral cavity also is moist, and membranes (including the lips) are smooth and intact.
B. Altered findings
1. Dry tongue with visible fissures or furrows
2. Dry membranes
3. Viscous mucus
4. Cracked and chapped lips
C. Possible causes of alterations
1. FVD due to conditions such as:
  a. Frank blood loss
  b. GI losses
  c. Excessive diuretic therapy
2. Hypernatremia due to conditions such as:
  a. Primary hyperaldosteronism
  b. Diabetes insipidus
  c. Burns

VII. Body weight

A. Normal findings

1. Total body weight (TBW) depends on the patient's height, sex, and bone structure.
2. Fluid status also plays a role in the determination of TBW. ECF represents approximately 20% of total body weight; ICF, approximately 40%.
3. One liter of fluid is approximately equivalent to 1 kg (2.2 lb) of TBW; therefore, the loss or gain of 1 kg of TBW indicates approximately 1 L of combined ECF and ICF fluid loss or gain.
4. In a healthy adult, TBW should remain relatively unchanged.
5. In a patient with third-space fluid shifting, weight gain may occur despite FVD in the intravascular space.

B. Altered findings

1. Rapid weight loss, ranging from 2% to 8% of TBW
2. Rapid weight gain, ranging from 2% to 8% of TBW

C. Possible causes of alterations

1. Rapid weight loss is associated with FVD and hypernatremia.
2. Rapid weight gain is associated with FVE, particularly conditions in which there is significant edema.

VIII. Thirst

A. Normal findings

1. The thirst center is located in the hypothalamus.
2. As fluid is lost, osmoreceptors shrink to stimulate thirst and increase oral intake.
3. As hydration status stabilizes, the water content of the osmoreceptors increases, and the thirst response is no longer experienced.

B. Altered findings

1. Increased oral intake due to the thirst response, despite normal hydration status
2. Poor oral intake despite subjective feelings of thirst

C. Possible causes of alterations

1. Neurologic disorders (eg, head trauma, malignancy, or vascular insult) have been known to cause hypothalamic injury, resulting in deficits in the thirst experience.
2. Psychogenic polydypsia is a psychologic disease that results in increased fluid intake despite normal hydration status.
3. Neuromuscular disease or coma result in the inability to take in fluids despite subjective feelings of thirst.

IX. Tearing and salivation

A. Normal findings

1. Tears are produced for the purpose of lubricating the eyes and thus protecting them from abrasions.
2. Salivation is stimulated by smells, thoughts, or the actual

presence of food; its purpose is to lubricate food to facilitate movement into the GI tract.

    B. **Altered findings**
        1. Decreased tearing
        2. Decreased salivation

    C. **Possible causes of alterations: Causes are the same as for alterations in tongue turgor and mucous membrane moisture (see Section VI.C).**

X. **Skin and body temperature**
    A. **Normal findings**
        1. Normal skin is warm and dry; skin color varies depending on perfusion, but generally it manifests with good turgor and appearance.
        2. Body temperature is approximately 98.6°F or 37°C; variations occur depending on the method of testing and individual idiosyncrasies.

    B. **Altered findings**
        1. Elevated skin and body temperature (occur as perspiration decreases and the body is less efficient in maintaining normothermia)
        2. Dry, flaky skin

    C. **Possible causes of alterations: Causes are the same as for alterations in tongue turgor and mucous membrane moisture (see Section VI.C).**

XI. **Edema**
    A. **Normal findings**
        1. A normal hydration status is not associated with edema.
        2. Skin is normally pliant with good elasticity, but no swelling is present.

    B. **Altered findings**
        1. Edema (deposition of fluid in the interstitial tissue)
        2. Pitting edema (severe interstitial fluid accumulation resulting in the tissue's inability to return to normal configuration after pressure is applied)

    C. **Possible causes of alterations**
        1. Peripheral dependent edema is caused by FVE.
        2. Edema also can result from vascular abnormalities and systemic conditions (eg, CHF).

XII. **Pulse**
    A. **Normal findings**
        1. The normal pulse is strong and regular.
        2. Heart rate is between 60 and 100 beats/min.

    B. **Altered findings**
        1. Bounding pulse
        2. Weak and thready pulse

        3. Bradycardia (< 60 beats/min)

        4. Tachycardia (> 100 beats/min)

C. Possible causes of alterations

        1. A bounding pulse is associated with FVE.

        2. A weak, thready pulse is associated with impending cardiovascular collapse; causes of cardiovascular collapse include:

            a. Severe FVD

            b. Hyperkalemia

            c. Hypocalcemia

            d. Hyperphosphatemia

        3. Bradycardia is associated with hypokalemia and hypermagnesemia.

        4. Tachycardia is associated with FVD (it occurs as a compensatory sympathetic nervous system response), respiratory acidosis, and hypernatremia.

        5. Pulse rate irregularities caused by dysrhythmias are associated with metabolic acidosis, metabolic alkalosis, respiratory alkalosis, hypophosphatemia, and hypercalcemia.

XIII. Respiration

A. Normal findings

        1. Normal respiratory rate is between 12 and 20 breaths per minute.

        2. Normal respiratory pattern is regular with bilateral chest expansion.

        3. Lung sounds are clear to auscultation.

B. Altered findings

        1. Altered respiratory patterns, including:

            a. Hyperventilation

            b. Hypoventilation

            c. Kussmaul's breathing

        2. Abnormal breaths sounds, such as crackles on auscultation

        3. Increased work of breathing, including dyspnea and dyspnea on exertion

C. Possible causes of alterations

        1. Hyperventilation is associated with hyperchloremia and respiratory alkalosis.

        2. Hypoventilation is associated with metabolic alkalosis, respiratory acidosis, hypokalemia, and hypermagnesemia.

        3. Kussmaul's breathing is associated with metabolic acidosis.

        4. Laryngeal stridor is associated with hypocalcemia and hyperphosphatemia.

        5. Crackles on auscultation and dyspnea are associated with FVE.

XIV. Blood pressure

A. Normal findings

        1. Blood pressure is considered within normal ranges if systolic does not exceed 140 mm Hg and diastolic does not exceed 90 mm Hg.

    2. The lower range of acceptable blood pressure includes a systolic of 80 mm Hg and a diastolic of 50 mm Hg.

B. Altered findings

    1. Hypertension (> 140/90 mm Hg)

    2. Hypotension (< 80/50 mm Hg)

    3. Postural hypotension (drop in systolic pressure due to orthostatic changes)

C. Possible causes of alterations

    1. Hypertension is associated with FVE and hypomagnesemia.

    2. Hypotension is associated with FVD, metabolic acidosis, respiratory alkalosis, and hypermagnesemia.

    3. Postural hypotension may be seen in FVD.

XV. Neck veins and central venous pressure (CVP)

A. Normal findings

    1. Venous pressure can be calculated by observing the external jugular veins; visualizing pulsations with measurement to the sternal angle affords an estimate of venous pressure.

    2. Normal venous pressure is 3 to 4 cm above the sternal angle.

    3. CVP may be measured directly using a catheter in the vena cava.

    4. Normal CVP reading ranges from 5 to 19 cm of water or 6 to 12 mm Hg.

B. Altered findings

    1. Flat or distended neck veins

    2. Elevated or below-normal CVP

C. Possible causes of alterations

    1. Neck vein distension and elevated CVP readings are associated with FVE.

    2. Flattened neck veins and low CVP readings are associated with FVD.

XVI. Neuromuscular irritability

A. Normal findings: Intact neurologic function (eg, normal cognitive, motor, and sensory findings)

B. Altered findings

    1. Cognitive changes, ranging from mild alterations (eg, restlessness, irritability, and decreased mentation) to severe alterations (eg, disorientation and coma)

    2. Motor dysfunction (eg, fatigue or muscle weakness); may be associated with lack of coordination or decreased reflex response

    3. Severe neuromuscular changes, such as tetany and carpopedal spasms associated with Chvostek's and Trousseau's signs (Fig. 14–1)

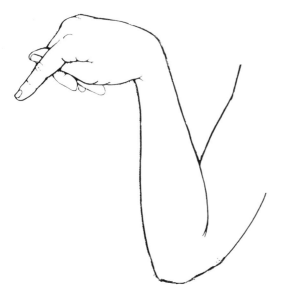

FIGURE 14–1.
Trousseau's sign. Carpopedal spasm with hypocalcemia.

4. Lack of coordination, such as is seen with vertigo, ataxia, and syncope
5. Sensory changes, including paresthesias, cramping, tetany, and Chvostek's and Trousseau's signs
6. Severe alterations (eg, seizures and psychoses)

C. **Possible causes of alterations**
   1. Cognitive changes have been associated with:
      a. FVD
      b. Acid–base imbalances
      c. Hypercalcemia
      d. Hypokalemia or hyperkalemia
      e. Hyponatremia or hypernatremia
      f. Hypochloremia or hyperchloremia
      g. Hypomagnesemia or hypermagnesemia
      h. Hypophosphatemia or hyperphosphatemia
   2. Neuromuscular alterations, such as weakness and tremors are associated with:
      a. Acid–base imbalances
      b. Alterations in potassium, calcium, sodium, magnesium, and chloride balance
   3. Tetany and hyperreflexia are associated with:
      a. Respiratory alkalosis
      b. Hypocalcemia
      c. Hypochloremia
      d. Hypomagnesemia
      e. Hyponatremia
      f. Hyperphosphatemia

    4. Weakness and hyporeflexia are associated with:
        a. Hypokalemia
        b. Hypophosphatemia
        c. Hypercalcemia
        d. Hypermagnesemia
    5. Sensory abnormalities, such as paresthesias, are associated with:
        a. Hypophosphatemia and hyperphosphatemia
        b. Hypomagnesemia
        c. Hyperkalemia
        d. Respiratory alkalosis

XVII. Nursing diagnoses

  A. **Overview of nursing diagnoses**

    1. Nursing diagnoses are conclusions derived from assessment findings; data from the patient history and examination are collected, analyzed, and synthesized. The result of that analysis is a nursing diagnosis.

    2. Accurate nursing diagnosis depends on accurate assessment; an assessment that does not include all necessary parameters will yield inaccurate data, which then yield an incorrect diagnosis.

    3. Nursing diagnoses affect implementation; incorrect diagnoses yield incorrect interventions, which result in poor patient outcomes.

    4. Diagnosing fluid, electrolyte, and acid–base imbalances requires a knowledge of pathophysiology, pharmacology, and fluid therapies and the ability to think critically:

        a. Knowledge of pathophysiology requires an understanding of how a particular disorder affects fluid, electrolyte, and acid–base balance in each patient.

        b. Knowledge of pharmacology requires an understanding how various drugs cause increases or decreases in fluid excretion or result in fluid and electrolyte shifts.

        c. Knowledge of fluid therapies requires an understanding of how parenteral therapies change the composition of body fluids and affect electrolyte status.

        d. Critical thinking allows the nurse to correctly analyze patient information and formulate an accurate nursing diagnosis.

    5. Nursing diagnoses for fluid, electrolyte, and acid–base imbalances affect all body systems.

  B. **Potential nursing diagnoses for fluid, electrolyte, and acid–base imbalances**

    1. Activity Intolerance
    2. Ineffective Airway Clearance

3. Anxiety
4. High Risk for Altered Body Temperature
5. Ineffective Breathing Pattern
6. Decreased Cardiac Output
7. Constipation
8. Diarrhea
9. Fatigue
10. Fluid Volume Deficit
11. Fluid Volume Excess
12. Impaired Gas Exchange
13. Altered Health Maintenance
14. Hyperthermia
15. Hypothermia
16. Altered Nutrition: Less than Body Requirements
17. Altered Oral Mucous Membranes
18. Pain
19. Impaired Skin Integrity
20. Impaired Tissue Perfusion
21. Urinary Elimination

Bibliography

Kinney M., Packa D., & Sunbar, S. (Eds.) (1993). *AACN's clinical reference for critical care nursing* (3rd ed.). St. Louis: C.V. Mosby.

Metheny, N. M. (1992). *Fluid and electrolyte balance: Nursing considerations* (2nd ed.). Philadelphia: J.B. Lippincott.

Thompson J., McFarland G., et al. (Eds.) (1993). *Clinical nursing* (3rd ed.). St. Louis: C.V. Mosby.

Bates, B. (1991). *A guide to physical examination and history taking* (5th ed.). Philadelphia: J.B. Lippincott.

STUDY QUESTIONS

1. The normal kidney maintains electrolyte and acid–base balance even when urine output is reduced to:
   a. 100 mL/day
   b. 10 mL/hour
   c. 500 mL/day
   d. 1000 mL/day

2. Which of the following findings would the nurse expect to assess in a patient with extrarenal fluid loss?
   a. hypothermia
   b. hypoventilation
   c. diarrhea
   d. distributive gain

3. Which of the following parameters provides information on urine concentration by measuring the total number of particles in solution?
   a. specific gravity
   b. urine osmolarity
   c. urine output
   d. BUN

4. Tachycardia is associated with fluid volume:
   a. deficits as a compensatory sympathetic nervous system response
   b. deficits related to hyponatremia
   c. excesses as a compensatory sympathetic nervous system response
   d. excesses related to fluid overload

5. A patient with chronic renal failure asks the nurse why his fluid intake is restricted. The nurse's best response would be:
   a. "Since your urine output is diminished, you can only ingest the amount you excrete."
   b. "Excessive free water intake will contribute to edema, because renal clearance is a concern."
   c. "Decreasing your oral intake will allow your kidneys to rest and heal."
   d. "Fluids are restricted because of your medication therapy."

6. In a patient with fluid volume excess (FVE), the neck veins appear to be:
   a. distended
   b. flattened
   c. retracted
   d. normal

7. During an examination, a patient exhibits hyperreflexia. The nurse knows that this is associated with:
   a. hypercalcemia
   b. hypermagnesemia
   c. respiratory acidosis
   d. hypocalcemia

8. When assessing a patient for fluid and electrolyte abnormalities, the nurse is aware that hypokalemia may cause:
   a. hyperreflexia
   b. paresthesia
   c. tetany
   d. hyporeflexia

ANSWER KEY

1. *Correct response: c*
   Because of its ability to concentrate fluids, the normal kidney can maintain electrolyte and acid–base balance even when urine output is reduced to 500 mL/day.
   a, b, and d. These responses are incorrect.
   Knowledge/Health promotion/Analysis

2. *Correct response: c*
   Extrarenal fluid loss refers to fluid loss that occurs in sites other than the kidney.
   a and b. Neither hypothermia nor hypoventilation cause fluid loss.
   d. This response is incorrect. It refers to a gain rather than a loss.
   Analysis/Health promotion/Assessment

3. *Correct response: b*
   Urine osmolarity is a measure of the total number of particles in solution, independent of size or weight.
   a. Specific gravity measures urine concentration but is dependent on the existence of solutes.
   c. Urine output does not provide information on urine concentration.
   d. BUN is a blood test.
   Comprehension/Physiologic/Assessment

4. *Correct response: a*
   Tachycardia is associated with fluid volume deficits as a compensatory sympathetic nervous system response.
   b, c, and d. These responses are incorrect.
   Comprehension/Physiologic/Assessment

5. *Correct response: b*
   In a patient with impaired renal clearance, excessive fluid intake can contribute to edema.
   a, c, and d. These responses are incorrect.
   Knowledge/Physiologic/Analysis

6. *Correct response: a*
   Neck veins are distended in FVE.
   b. Flattened neck veins occur in FVD.
   c. There is no such entity as retracted neck veins.
   d. Normal neck veins exist when normal fluid balance is present.
   Knowledge/Safe care/Assessment

7. *Correct response: d*
   Hyperreflexia is associated with hypocalcemia.
   a. This response is incorrect.
   b and c. Hypomagnesemia and respiratory alkalosis are associated with hyperreflexia.
   Application/Safe care/Assessment

8. *Correct response: d*
   Hyporeflexia and weakness are associated with hypokalemia.
   a and c. Tetany and hyperreflexia are not associated with fluctuating potassium levels.
   b. Paresthesias are associated with hyperkalemia.
   Comprehension/Safe care/Assessment

Disorders Associated With High Risk for Fluid, Electrolyte, and Acid–Base Imbalances

Paradiso, C: *Lippincott's Review Series: Fluids and Electrolytes* © 1995 J. B. Lippincott Company

B. Etiology
C. Pathophysiologic processes and clinical manifestations
D. Overview of nursing interventions

Bibliography
Study Questions

I. Introduction

A. Overview of imbalances
 1. Fluid and electrolyte deficiencies tend to be caused by conditions associated with:
  a. Decreased intake
  b. Excessive elimination
 2. Fluid and electrolyte excesses tend to be caused by conditions associated with:
  a. Excessive intake
  b. Decreased elimination
 3. Acid–base imbalances may be caused by metabolic conditions that affect regulatory mechanisms.

B. Types of disorders associated with imbalances
 1. Endocrine disorders in which protein, carbohydrate, or fat metabolism is altered, such as in:
  a. Diabetes insipidus
  b. Syndrome of inappropriate antidiuretic hormone (SIADH)
  c. Diabetic ketoacidosis (DKA)
  d. Hyperglycemic hyperosmolar nonketotic coma (HHNC)
 2. Renal disorders in which the buffer systems are inadequate or not functioning
 3. Gastrointestinal (GI) fluid losses due to altered metabolism or elimination
 4. Respiratory disorders
 5. Disorders of decreased cardiac output
 6. Burns
 7. Cirrhosis

II. Diabetes insipidus (DI)

A. Description and etiology
 1. DI is caused by inadequate secretion of antidiuretic hormone (ADH) from the pituitary gland; this may result from:
  a. Head trauma

        b.   Cerebral ischemia due to a cerebrovascular accident (CVA)

        c.   Pituitary or brain surgery

        d.   Endocrine disorders

    2.   ADH insufficiency reduces the amount of water eliminated in the kidney tubules, increasing urine volume and decreasing extracellular fluid (ECF) volume.

B.   **Pathophysiologic processes and clinical manifestions**

    1.   As a result of damage to the hypothalamus, the stalk, or the pituitary gland, insufficient amounts of ADH are released.

    2.   Lack of ADH allows excessive renal excretion of water, with liters being excreted each hour.

    3.   This excessive diuresis results in extracellular fluid volume deficit, which causes hypotension.

    4.   Because water is excreted in excess of sodium, hypernatremia occurs.

C.   **Overview of nursing interventions**

    1.   Administer replacement fluids as prescribed.

    2.   Monitor for hypotension and cardiovascular collapse.

    3.   Monitor electrolyte levels.

III. SIADH

A.   **Description**

    1.   SIADH involves continuous pituitary secretion of ADH when plasma osmolarity is low.

    2.   This hormonal excess increases the amount of water absorbed by the kidney tubules, decreasing urine volume and resulting in extracellular fluid volume excess (FVE).

B.   **Etiology**

    1.   Head trauma

    2.   Cerebral ischemia due to CVA

    3.   Endocrine disorders (eg, hyperpituitarism)

    4.   Pulmonary tumors in which the tumor secretes a chemical similar to ADH

    5.   Medications such as Dilantin

    6.   Brain surgery in which cerebral edema affects hormonal secretion

C.   **Pathophysiologic processes and clinical manifestions**

    1.   As a result of damage to either the hypothalamic messenger–releasing process or the pituitary gland, excessive amounts of ADH are secreted.

    2.   This excess is continuous and unregulated by the usual feedback mechanism.

    3.   ADH acts on the distal tubules to reabsorb water; excessive ADH secretion causes excessive water retention, diluting the ECF.

    4. This water retention causes osmolality to drop as particles are diluted, lowering serum osmolality and elevating urine osmolality.

    5. Excessive water retention also causes increased intravascular volume and increased blood pressure, inhibiting secretion of renin and aldosterone.

    6. Aldosterone inhibition reduces sodium absorption, causing hyponatremia through sodium loss. Excessive water retention dilutes sodium, also causing hyponatremia.

    7. The resulting hyponatremia is profound and life-threatening.

D. Overview of nursing interventions

    1. Measure and record carefully daily intake and output and weight.

    2. Restrict water intake.

    3. Monitor vital signs frequently.

    4. Monitor serum sodium concentration closely because the cells can become water logged, altering the patient's sensorium.

    5. Administer hypertonic saline as ordered if hyponatremia is severe:

        a. Give hypertonic saline *with caution* because a rapid shift of water from the ICF to ECF can result in congestive heart failure (CHF).

        b. Administer Lasix with the hypertonic saline as ordered to eliminate excess water shifting into the ECF.

IV. DKA

A. Description

    1. DKA is a condition characterized by acute insulin deficiency, resulting in metabolic acidosis due to the presence of ketone bodies.

    2. It commonly occurs in patients with undiagnosed diabetes.

B. Etiology

    1. Insufficient insulin secretion

    2. Inadequate insulin intake (possibly due to the patient's failure to take insulin as prescribed)

    3. Stressful situations (eg, surgery, infection, emotional stress, trauma) in which steroid hormones are secreted; these hormones act as antagonists to insulin, causing glucose levels to rise.

C. Pathophysiologic processes and clinical manifestations

    1. As glucose levels rise, hyperglycemia occurs as a lack of insulin prevents use of glucose, the body's primary energy source.

    2. As a result, the body burns fat, its secondary energy source.

    3. Fat metabolism yields ketone bodies as an acid end-product, resulting in metabolic acidosis.

    4. The respiratory system tries to compensate for the increased

acids through deep, rapid breathing known as Kussmaul's respirations.

5. The body tries to eliminate the excess acids by increasing acid excretion, causing ketonuria; ketones also are present in the serum.

6. The large amount of glucose present in the serum causes hyperosmolality, which produces osmotic diuresis (because glucose tends to attract water); osmotic diuresis contributes to hyponatremia and may cause fluid and electrolyte losses.

7. As fluid is eliminated from the intravascular space through the urine, dehydration may result and electrolyte shifts may occur.

8. Hypokalemia occurs as osmotic diuresis promotes potassium excretion and acidemia shifts potassium out of the cells.

9. In response to fluid loss, aldosterone is secreted, causing sodium reabsorption and potassium elimination and further exacerbation of hypokalemia.

10. In response to hyperglycemia, potassium moves from the ECF to the ICF.

D. Overview of nursing interventions

1. Administer regular insulin to decrease serum glucose as ordered; monitor serum glucose levels to avoid overcorrection and hypoglycemia.

2. Administer bicarbonate as ordered if acidosis is severe.

3. Monitor serum potassium as potassium moves from the ICF to the ECF during correction of acidosis.

4. Rehydrate patient as ordered with 0.9% sodium chloride or lactated Ringer's solution; be aware that replacement may need to be rapid (eg, as much as 1 L/h).

6. Assess fluid volume status, and maintain blood pressure.

7. Measure and record carefully intake and output; insert a Foley catheter to obtain hourly measurements.

8. Monitor hemodynamic parameters.

9. Measure weight daily.

10. Monitor arterial blood gases (ABGs), electrolyte levels, and serum osmolality.

V. HHNC

A. Description

1. HHNC is characterized by a relative insulin deficiency (as opposed to DKA, in which an absolute insulin deficiency exists).

2. In HHNC, enough insulin is present to spare the body from accelerated fat metabolism; the result is hyperglycemia without ketonuria.

3. HHNC commonly occurs in patients with undiagnosed diabetes or in middle-aged patients with non–insulin-dependent diabetes mellitus.

B. Etiology
1. Inadequate insulin secretion or action
2. Unintentional dietary indiscretions (eg, inadequate insulin intake)
3. Ingestion of certain medications (eg, thiazide diuretics, glucocorticoids, phenytoin, sympathomimetics)

C. Pathophysiologic processes and clinical manifestions
1. Not enough insulin is present to prevent hyperglycemia; however, enough is present to prevent ketonuria.
2. As a result of high serum glucose levels, glycosuria and polyuria from osmotic diuresis occur.
3. Polyuria results in dehydration of the ECF and ICF, causing neurologic changes.

D. Overview of nursing interventions
1. Monitor vital signs.
2. Measure and record intake and output.
3. Assess fluid and electrolyte status.

VI. Renal disease

A. Description
1. Renal disease may be acute or chronic:
   a. Acute disease occurs suddenly and typically is reversible.
   b. Chronic disease develops over a longer period of time and often is not reversible.
2. Renal diseases that can cause fluid and electrolyte imbalances include:
   a. Acute or chronic renal failure
   b. Acute tubular necrosis
   c. Pyelonephritis and glomerulonephritis
   d. Obstructive disorders (eg, stones, tumors)

B. Etiology
1. Insufficient renal blood flow
2. Damage to the renal parenchyma
3. Administration of nephrotoxins
4. Infectious agents

C. Pathophysiologic processes and clinical manifestions
1. When the kidneys fail, no mechanism for maintaining fluid, electrolyte, and acid–base balance exists.
2. Depending on the mechanism of failure, damage occurs to the glomerulus or tubules, or both:
   a. Damage to the glomerulus hinders filtration capabilities, allowing excess fluids and electrolytes to pass.
   b. Damage to the tubules causes them to become more or less permeable, resulting in altered elimination patterns.

3. Damage to the glomerulus and filter also causes the buffer systems (protein, phosphate, bicarbonate) to fail, altering acid–base balance.
4. Kidney damage also alters hormone secreting capabilities, affecting the levels of renin and erythropoietin:
   a. Oversecretion of renin commonly occurs in renal failure, resulting in high blood pressure.
   b. Inadequate erythropoietin secretion contributed to anemia before the hormone was available by parenteral preparation (Epogen).
5. As acid waste products accumulate, they are unable to be buffered because the buffering mechanisms have failed.
6. In low output states, fluid and electrolyte imbalances occur; these can include:
   a. Hypervolemia
   b. Hypernatremia
   c. Hyperkalemia
   d. Hypocalcemia
   e. Hyperphosphatemia
   f. Hypermagnesemia
   g. Metabolic acidosis
7. Hypervolemia can result in CHF or pulmonary edema.
8. If the kidneys are not adequately perfused with blood, the nephrons will be damaged; as a result, the cause may be hard to distinguish from the effect if only output is evaluated.

D. Overview of nursing interventions
1. Maintain accurate assessment of fluid balance by measuring and recording daily weights and intake and output and by closely monitoring vital signs, breath sounds, and hemodynamic parameters (if available).
2. Be aware of signs of fluid overload (eg, dyspnea, rales, bounding pulse, edema, bulging neck veins).
3. Monitor electrolyte levels because some electrolyte imbalances have deleterious effects.
4. Monitor ABGs.
5. Monitor electrocardiogram changes because disorders of potassium and calcium can cause cardiac dysrhythmias.
6. Maintain dietary restrictions.
7. Administer diuretics as ordered if the patient's kidneys are still able to eliminate urine.
8. Administer bicarbonate as ordered if acidosis is severe; be aware that this may cause hypocalcemia because bicarbonate tends to bind calcium.
9. Initiate dialysis if necessary.

VII.   GI fluid losses

  A.   Description: Excessive fluid losses (eg, intestinal secretions, gastric fluid, pancreatic juice) through the upper or lower GI tract

  B.   Etiology

   1.   Viral or bacterial infection

   2.   Ulcers

   3.   Inflammatory diseases

   4.   Obstructions

   5.   Surgical tubes

   6.   Vomiting

   7.   Tube drainage

  C.   Pathophysiologic processes and clinical manifestations

   1.   The types of fluid and electrolyte disorders that result from GI fluid losses depend on the amount and type of fluid lost.

   2.   Because fluids in the upper GI tract (eg, stomach, intestine, and pancreas) are rich in sodium, potassium, chloride, and hydrogen, upper GI losses tend to cause hypokalemia and metabolic alkalosis from loss of hydrogen.

   3.   Fluids in the lower GI tract are alkaline; as a result, acidosis commonly occurs when bases are lost due to diarrhea, fistulas, and ileostomies.

  D.   Overview of nursing interventions

   1.   Measure and record intake and output carefully to track fluid losses.

   2.   Administer replacement solutions as ordered.

   3.   Assess fluid and electrolyte status.

   4.   Monitor ABGs.

   5.   Administer medications (eg, histamine 2-receptor antagonists, antacids, losec) as ordered.

VIII.   Respiratory dysfunction

  A.   Description and etiology

   1.   The lungs play a critical role in maintaining the balance of CO_2 an acid.

   2.   Changes in the respiratory volume and rate (eg, hypoventilation or hyperventilation) alter the amount of CO_2 that is retained or excreted, resulting in respiratory acidosis or respiratory alkalosis.

   3.   Hypoventilation may result from:

      a.   Central nervous system disorders (eg, stroke, head injury) in which the central stimulus to breathe is reduced by damage to the brain

      b.   Respiratory disorders involving obstruction or fluid accumulation (eg, chronic obstructive pulmonary disorder, tumors, pulmonary edema, pneumonia)

      c.   Cardiac disorders (eg, CHF)

    4. Hyperventilation may result from:
       a. Tachypnea
       b. Inappropriate mechanical ventilation settings

B. **Pathophysiologic processes and clinical manifestations**
    1. *Hypoventilation* reduces oxygen delivery to the alveoli and CO_2 elimination, allowing retention of the acid CO_2.
    2. As a result, respiratory acidosis occurs; ABG values reflect a low pH and a high CO_2.
    3. *Hyperventilation* results in excess CO_2 elimination, leaving excess base (bicarbonate) in the blood and resulting in respiratory alkalosis; ABG values reflect high pH and low CO_2.
    4. Patients who are mechanically ventilated may be hyperventilated or hypoventilated by inappropriate ventilator settings.

C. **Overview of nursing interventions**
    1. Monitor ABGs.
    2. Assess respiratory status.
    3. Administer oxygen as prescribed.
    4. Administer treatments to correct the cause of acidosis or alkalosis.

IX. **Decreased cardiac output**

A. **Description: Inability of the heart to pump enough blood to perfuse the tissues and vital organs adequately; renal hypoperfusion results in FVE.**

B. **Etiology**
    1. CHF (may occur from volume expansion or pump failure)
    2. Cardiac depressant medication (eg, anesthetics)
    3. Cardiomyopathy
    4. Volume expansion
    5. Myocardial infarction

C. **Pathophysiologic processes and clinical manifestations**
    1. As the heart's pumping ability fails, blood is unable to be ejected from the right ventricle to the lungs or from the left ventricle to the periphery.
    2. The blood vessels then lose pressure (hypotension) because the pumping force is inadequate to propel the blood.
    3. Renal hypoperfusion, which can eventually cause prerenal azotemia, is sensed in the juxtaglomerular cells; in response, these cells secrete renin.
    4. The renin-angiotensin-aldosterone mechanism allows excess sodium to be reabsorbed in the kidney tubules.
    5. This sodium reabsorption also is accompanied by water reabsorption, exacerbating FVE.
    6. Angiotensin causes massive vasoconstriction, forcing the heart to pump against the increased pressure, adding to afterload and exacerbating heart failure.

7. Total congestion of the heart's right or left side, or both sides, occurs.

8. In right-sided heart failure, the ventricle is unable to eject blood into the aorta and through to the peripheral tissues; blood then backs up into the left atrium, pulmonary veins, and the pulmonary vasculature. Symptoms of right-sided heart failure include edema of the organs (eg, liver) and periphery (eg, feet, legs, and sacrum).

9. In left-sided heart failure, the left ventricle is unable to eject blood from itself into the lungs; blood then backs up into the atrium, vena cava, and periphery. Symptoms of left-sided heart failure include manifestations of pulmonary edema:

   a. Rales at the bases
   b. Tachycardia
   c. Hypoxia (due to pulmonary fluid accumulation)
   d. Restlessness, diaphoresis, orthopnea, anuria, excessive pink secretions (these occur in the late stages)

10. If hypoperfusion is severe, metabolic acidosis results from excess lactic acid accumulation.

D. Overview of nursing interventions

1. Monitor fluid and electrolyte balance.
2. Monitor vital signs and hemodynamic parameters.
3. Provide a low-sodium diet.
4. Monitor pulmonary status closely, because life-threatening pulmonary edema can result.
5. Monitor serum electrolyte levels and ABGs.
6. Administer medications as prescribed to improve cardiac output.

X. Burns

A. Description and etiology

1. Burns are traumatic injuries to the skin resulting from heat, electrical current, chemicals, friction, shearing forces, or excessive exposure to sunlight.
2. Burns are classified according to the depth of destruction to the epidermis, dermis, or subcutaneous layers:

   a. *First-degree burn* (partial thickness)
   b. *Second-degree burn* (superficial or deep partial thickness)
   c. *Third-degree burn* (full thickness)

B. Pathophysiologic processes and clinical manifestations

1. When the skin is burned, body fluids and electrolytes leak out.
2. The type and severity of the resultant fluid and electrolyte disorders depend on the extent of the burn; typically, severe burns pose the highest risk for significant disorders.
3. After a severe burn, edema accounts for some loss of plasma

volume as fluid moves from the intravascular to the interstitial space and eventually to the intracellular space.

4. Water evaporation also occurs, further exacerbating fluid loss; this insensible loss cannot be measured and may be severe.

5. As plasma volume is lost, blood pressure drops, leading to poor perfusion of vital organs. Proteins and electrolytes also are lost. Blood loss may occur as well.

6. Decreased tissue perfusion produces lactic acid, causing metabolic acidosis.

7. Hypoventilation results in CO_2 retention, causing respiratory acidosis.

8. Because potassium is released whenever cells are destroyed, hyperkalemia can occur; it worsens if the burn is complicated by renal failure.

9. After 4 to 5 days, potassium may shift from the ECF to the ICF; extracellular FVE occurs as fluid shifts from the interstitial space into the intravascular space.

10. Hyponatremia occurs as large amounts of sodium are trapped in edema fluid. It also may result as fluids are remobilized.

D. **Overview of nursing interventions**

1. Administer IV fluid replacement therapy as ordered to restore depleted volume.

2. Assess cardiac, pulmonary, and fluid volume status.

3. Assess hemodynamic measurements to track the effectiveness of fluid volume replacement therapy.

4. Maintain patent airway if the upper airway is damaged from smoke inhalation.

XI. Cirrhosis

A. **Description**

1. Cirrhosis is an irreversible chronic inflammatory disease characterized by massive degeneration and destruction of hepatocytes, resulting in a disorganized lobular pattern of regeneration.

2. Classifications of cirrhosis based on morphologic changes in regenerated nodules include micronodular cirrhosis, macronodular cirrhosis, and mixed cirrhosis.

B. **Etiology**

1. Alcoholism
2. Hepatotoxic medications
3. Blood transfusion reaction
4. Poor cardiac perfusion (right-sided CHF)
5. Biliary tract obstruction (strictures)
6. Complication of hepatitis

C. **Pathophysiologic processes and clinical manifestations**

1. Cirrhosis is a complicated disease, but it affects fluid and elec-

trolyte balance in that liver damage prevents aldosterone and other hormones from metabolizing.

2. The presence of aldosterone leads to increased sodium reabsorption and subsequent potassium elimination (in some cases).

3. Water is reabsorbed along with sodium; the excess sodium and water tend to accumulate in the feet as pedal edema and in the abdomen as ascites.

4. Ascites results because of the poor metabolism of protein; when protein is present in the abdominal circulation as the blood exits the liver, it exerts its osmotic effect by drawing fluid into the peritoneal cavity.

D. Overview of nursing interventions

1. Administer spironolactone (Aldactone) as ordered to inhibit the sodium-retaining action of aldosterone; because sodium excretion is now possible, potassium will be retained, making hyperkalemia a possible complication.

2. Monitor the patient's amount of dietary protein intake, because patients with cirrhosis need more protein than others.

3. Measure abdominal girth daily to track the amount of fluid retained.

4. Monitor daily intake and output.

5. Measure and record daily weight.

6. Assess the patient for changes in cardiac output, decreased renal function, and electrolyte imbalances.

Bibliography

Alspach, J. G. (1991). *Core curriculum for critical care nursing* (4th ed.). Philadelphia: W.B. Saunders.

Brunner, L. S., & Suddarth, D. S. (1992). *Textbook of medical-surgical nursing* (7th ed.). Philadelphia: J.B. Lippincott.

Guyton, A. (1991). *Textbook of medical physiology* (8th ed.). Philadelphia: W.B. Saunders.

McCance, K. L., & Huether, S. E. (1994). *Pathophysiology: The biologic basis for disease in adults and children* (2nd ed.). St. Louis: Mosby–Year Book.

Metheny, N. (1992). *Fluid and electrolyte balance: Nursing considerations* (2nd ed.). Philadelphia: J.B. Lippincott.

STUDY QUESTIONS

1. The mechanism by which hypoventilation results in acidosis involves:
   a. excretion of the acid CO_2
   b. retention of the acid CO_2
   c. retention of oxygen
   d. excretion of oxygen

2. The nurse would interpret a blood gas pH of 7.30 as indicating:
   a. acidosis
   b. alkalosis
   c. normal
   d. hypoxia

3. When assessing a patient with congestive heart failure (CHF), the nurse is aware that symptoms of left-sided heart failure include:
   a. sacral edema
   b. liver edema
   c. rales at the bases
   d. pedal edema

4. The nurse has provided patient teaching about dietary modifications for a patient with CHF. Which of the following menu selections indicates that the patient needs further education?
   a. corned beef sandwich
   b. fruit salad
   c. tuna salad sandwich
   d. bagel with butter

5. Nursing management of CHF includes:
   a. encouraging fluids
   b. keeping the head of the bed flat
   c. encouraging ambulation
   d. administering diuretics as ordered

6. Which of the following nursing diagnoses is consistent with diabetes insipidus?
   a. extracellular fluid volume deficit (FVD)
   b. intracellular fluid volume excess (FVE)
   c. extracellular FVE
   d. intracellular FVD

7. Metabolic acidosis occurs in diabetic ketoacidosis because:
   a. Aldosterone is an acid that is released.
   b. Lack of sugar causes acid release.
   c. Fat metabolism yields acid ketone bodies.
   d. Hyperventilation causes acid retention.

8. When estimating fluid loss, the nurse knows that fluid and electrolyte losses from severe burns occur through the skin and:
   a. blood vessels from bleeding
   b. fluid shifting and evaporation
   c. vomiting and diarrhea from shock
   d. all of the above

9. Which of the following acid–base imbalances is associated with burns?
   a. respiratory acidosis
   b. metabolic acidosis
   c. respiratory alkalosis
   d. metabolic alkalosis

ANSWER KEY

1. **Correct response: b**
Hypoventilation reduces oxygen delivery to the alveoli and carbon dioxide elimination, allowing for retention of the acid CO_2 and acidosis.
a, c, and d. These responses are incorrect.
Comprehension/Safe care/Analysis

2. **Correct response: a**
A pH lower then 7.35 indicates acidosis.
b. A pH greater than 7.45 indicates alkalosis
c. Normal pH is 7.35–7.45.
d. This response is incorrect.
Knowledge/Physiologic/Assessment

3. **Correct response: c**
In left-sided CHF, fluid backs up into the lungs; symptoms include rales at the bases and hypoxia.
a, b, and d. These are symptoms of right-sided CHF.
Comprehension/Safe care/Assessment

4. **Correct response: a**
Corned beef contains high amounts of sodium, as do other smoked and preserved meats.
b, c, and d. These would be better menu selections.
Analysis/Safe care/Implementation

5. **Correct response: d**
Treatment for a patient with CHF involves administering digoxin and diuretics, providing a low-sodium diet, keeping the head of the bed elevated, and encouraging bedrest.
a, b, and c. These are contraindicated in CHF.
Comprehension/Safe care/Implementation

6. **Correct response: a**
Lack of antidiuretic hormone (ADH) allows excessive renal excretion of water, with liters being excreted each hour.
b. Intracellular FVE would be associated with a condition that produced sodium losses in excess of water.
c. Extracellular FVE would be associated with a gain of water and salt.
d. Intracellular FVD would be associated with a gain of hypertonic solutions.
Comprehension/Physiologic/Analysis (Dx)

7. **Correct response: c**
Fat metabolism yields ketone bodies as an acid end-product, resulting in metabolic acidosis; fat metabolism occurs as the body uses fat for energy.
a. Aldosterone is a hormone, not an acid.
b. This response in incorrect.
d. Hyperventilation causes acid diminution, *not* retention.
Comprehension/Physiologic/NA

8. **Correct response: b**
After a severe burn injury, edema accounts for some loss of plasma volume as fluid shifts occur. Water evaporation also occurs, increasing insensible fluid loss. Fluid shifting must always be accounted for when calculating fluid loss.
a and c. Fluid and electrolyte loss may occur via these routes, but not always.
d. This response is incorrect.
Comprehension/Physiologic/NA

9. **Correct response: b**
Metabolic acidosis results as decreased tissue perfusion produces lactic acidosis.
a, c, and d. These acid–base disorders are not necessarily associated with burns.
Knowledge/Physiologic/NA

COMPREHENSIVE TEST QUESTIONS

1. The nurse would interpret a serum chloride level of 96 mEq/L as:
   a. high
   b. low
   c. within normal range
   d. high normal

2. Which of the following conditions is *not* associated with elevated serum chloride levels?
   a. nephritis
   b. diabetes
   c. eclampsia
   d. cardiac disease

3. In the extracellular fluid, chloride is a major:
   a. compound
   b. ion
   c. anion
   d. cation

4. Nursing interventions for the patient with hyperphosphatemia include encouraging intake of:
   a. Amphojel
   b. Fleet's phospho-soda
   c. milk
   e. vitamin D

5. Etiologies associated with hypocalcemia may include all of the following *except:*
   a. renal failure
   b. inadequate intake calcium
   c. metastatic bone lesions
   d. vitamin D deficiency

6. Which of the following findings would the nurse expect to assess in hypercalcemia?
   a. prolonged QRS complex
   b. tetany
   c. petechiae
   d. urinary calculi

7. Which of the following is not an appropriate nursing intervention for a patient with hypercalcemia?
   a. administering calcitonin
   b. administering calcium gluconate

   c. administering loop diuretics
   d. encouraging ambulation

8. A patient with which of the following disorders is at high risk to develop hypermagnesemia?
   a. insulin shock
   b. hyperadrenalism
   c. nausea and vomiting
   d. renal failure

9. Nursing interventions for a patient with hypermagnesemia include administering calcium gluconate to:
   a. increase calcium levels
   b. antagonize the cardiac effects of magnesium
   c. lower calcium levels
   d. lower magnesium levels

10. For a patient with hypomagnesemia, which of the following medications may become toxic?
    a. Lasix
    b. Digoxin
    c. calcium gluconate
    d. CAPD

11. Which of the following is *not* a physical assessment parameter the nurse would consider when assessing fluid and electrolyte balance?
    a. skin turgor
    b. intake and output
    c. osmotic pressure
    d. blood pressure, pulse, and central venous pressure

12. Insensible fluid losses include:
    a. urine
    b. gastric drainage
    c. bleeding
    d. perspiration

13. Which of the following intravenous solutions would be appropriate for a patient with severe hyponatremia secondary to syndrome of inappropriate antidiuretic hormone (SIADH)?
    a. hypotonic solution
    b. hypertonic solution

c. isotonic solution
d. normotonic solution

14. Aldosterone secretion in response to fluid loss will result in which one of the following electrolyte imbalances?
a. hypokalemia
b. hyperkalemia
c. hyponatremia
d. hypernatremia

15. When assessing a patient for signs of fluid overload, the nurse would *not* expect to observe:
a. bounding pulse
b. bulging neck veins
c. poor skin turgor
d. rales

16. The physician has ordered IV replacement of potassium for a patient with severe hypokalemia. The nurse would administer this:
a. by rapid bolus
b. diluted in 100 mL over 1 hour
c. diluted in 10 mL over 10 minutes
d. IV push

17. Which of the following findings would the nurse expect to assess in a patient with hypokalemia?
a. hypertension
b. pH below 7.35
c. hypoglycemia
d. hyporeflexia

18. Oral potassium supplements should be administered:
a. undiluted
b. diluted
c. on an empty stomach
d. at bedtime

19. Normal venous blood pH ranges from:
a. 6.8 to 7.2
b. 7.31 to 7.41
c. 7.35 to 7.45
d. 7.0 to 8.0

20. Respiratory regulation of acids and bases involves:
a. hydrogen
b. hydroxide
c. oxygen
d. carbon dioxide

21. To determine if a patient's respiratory system is functioning, the nurse would assess all of the following parameters *except:*
a. respiratory rate
b. respiratory depth
c. arterial blood gas
d. pulse oximetry

22. Which of the following conditions is an equal decrease of extracellular fluid (ECF) solute and water volume?
a. hypotonic FVD
b. isotonic FVD
c. hypertonic FVD
d. isotonic FVE

23. When monitoring the daily weight of a patient with fluid volume deficit (FVD), the nurse is aware that fluid loss may be considered when weight loss begins to exceed:
a. 0.25 lb
b. 0.50 lb
c. 1 lb
d. 1 kg

24. Dietary recommendations for a patient with a hypotonic fluid excess should include:
a. decreased sodium intake
b. increased sodium intake
c. increased fluid intake
d. intake of potassium-rich foods

25. Osmotic pressure is created through the process of:
a. osmosis
b. diffusion
c. filtration
d. capillary dynamics

26. A rise in arterial pressure causes the baroreceptors and stretch receptors to signal an inhibition of the sympathetic nervous system, resulting in:
a. decreased sodium reabsorption
b. increased sodium reabsorption
c. decreased urine output
d. increased urine output

27. Normal serum sodium concentration ranges from:
a. 120 to 125 mEq/liter
b. 125 to 130 mEq/liter

c. 136 to 145 mEq/liter
d. 140 to 148 mEq/liter

28. When assessing a patient for electrolyte balance, the nurse is aware that
etiologies for hyponatremia include all
of the following *except:*
   a. water gain
   b. diuretic therapy
   c. diaphoresis
   d. water loss

29. Nursing interventions for a patient
with hyponatremia include:
   a. administering hypotonic IV fluids
   b. encouraging water intake
   c. restricting fluid intake
   d. restricting sodium intake

30. The nurse would analyze an arterial
pH of 7.46 as indicating:
   a. acidosis
   b. alkalosis
   c. homeostasis
   d. neutrality

31. The net diffusion of water from one
solution through a semipermeable
membrane to another solution containing a lower concentration of water
is termed:
   a. filtration
   b. diffusion
   c. osmosis
   d. brownian motion

32. When assessing a patient's total body
water percentage, the nurse is aware
that all of the following factors influence this *except:*
   a. age
   b. fat tissue
   c. muscle mass
   d. sex

33. Which of the following symptoms
would the nurse expect to assess in a
patient with fluid volume deficit
(FVD)?
   a. rales
   b. bounding pulse
   c. tachycardia
   d. bulging neck veins

34. Nursing management of a patient receiving hypertonic fluids includes

monitoring for all of the following potential complications *except:*
   a. water intoxication
   b. fluid volume excess (FVE)
   c. cellular dehydration
   d. cell shrinkage

35. A patient is scheduled to receive an
isotonic solution; which one of the
following solutions is *not* isotonic?
   a. 0.33% saline
   b. 0.45% saline
   c. 0.9% saline
   d. D_5W

36. Which of the following arterial blood
gas (ABG) values indicates uncompensated metabolic alkalosis?
   a. pH 7.48, $PaCO_2$ 42, HCO_3 30
   b. pH 7.48, $PaCO_2$ 46, HCO_3 30
   c. pH 7.48, $PaCO_2$ 34, HCO_3 20
   d. pH 7.48, $PaCO_2$ 34, HCO_3 26

37. The body's compensation of metabolic alkalosis involves:
   a. increasing the respiratory rate
   b. decreasing the respiratory rate
   c. increasing urine output
   d. decreasing urine output

38. When assessing a patient for metabolic
alkalosis, the nurse would *not* expect
to assess:
   a. low serum potassium
   b. increased respiratory rate
   c. paresthesias
   d. stupor

39. Which of the following blood products should be infused rapidly?
   a. packed red blood cells (PRBC)
   b. fresh frozen plasma (FFP)
   c. platelets
   d. dextran

40. Which of the following statements
provides the rationale for using a hypotonic solution for a patient with
FVD?
   a. A hypotonic solution provides free
water to help the kidneys eliminate the solute.
   b. A hypotonic solution supplies an
excess of sodium and chloride ions.
   c. Excessive volumes are recom-

mended in the early postoperative period.

d. A hypotonic solution is used to treat hyponatremia.

41. When monitoring a patient who is receiving a blood transfusion, the nurse would analyze an elevated body temperature as indicating:
a. a normal physiologic process
b. evidence of sepsis
c. a possible transfusion reaction
d. an expected response to the transfusion

42. The process of endocrine regulation of electrolytes involves:
a. sodium reabsorption and chloride excretion
b. chloride reabsorption and sodium excretion
c. potassium reabsorption and sodium excretion
d. sodium reabsorption and potassium excretion

43. The chief anion in the intracellular fluid (ICF) is:
a. phosphorus
b. potassium
c. sodium
d. chloride

44. The major cation in the ICF is:
a. potassium
b. sodium
c. phosphorus
d. magnesium

45. Hypophosphatemia may result from which of the following diseases?
a. liver cirrhosis
b. renal failure
c. Paget's disease
d. alcoholism

46. A patient with which of the following disorders is at high risk for developing hyperphosphatemia?
a. hyperkalemia
b. hyponatremia
c. hypocalcemia
d. hyperglycemia

47. Normal calcium levels must be analyzed in relation to

a. sodium
b. glucose
c. protein
d. fats

48. Calcium is absorbed in the GI tract under the influence of:
a. vitamin D
b. glucose
c. HCl
d. vitamin C

49. Which of the following nursing diagnoses is most appropriate for a patient with hypocalcemia?
a. Constipation, Bowel
b. High Risk for Injury: Bleeding
c. Airway Clearance, Ineffective
d. High Risk for Injury: Confusion

50. When serum calcium levels rise, which of the following hormones is secreted?
a. aldosterone
b. renin
c. parathyroid hormone
d. calcitonin

51. The presence of which of the following electrolytes contributes to acidosis?
a. sodium
b. potassium
c. hydrogen
d. chloride

52. The lungs participate in acid–base balance by:
a. reabsorbing bicarbonate
b. splitting carbonic acid in two
c. using CO_2 to regulate hydrogen ions
d. sending hydrogen ions to the renal tubules

53. The respiratory system regulates acid–base balance by:
a. increasing mucus production
b. changing the rate and depth of respirations
c. forming bicarbonate
d. reabsorbing bicarbonate

54. Which of the following is a gas component of the ABG measurement?
a. carbon dioxide
b. bicarbonate

c. hydrogen

d. pH

55. Chloride helps maintain acid–base balance by performing which of the following roles?

   a. participating in the chloride shift

   b. following sodium to maintain serum osmolarity

   c. maintaining the balance of cations in the ICF and ECF

   d. separating carbonic acid

56. Which of the following hormones helps regulate chloride reabsorption?

   a. antidiuretic hormone (ADH)

   b. renin

   c. estrogen

   d. aldosterone

57. Chloride is absorbed in the:

   a. stomach

   b. bowel

   c. liver

   d. kidney

58. When chloride concentration drops below 95 mEq/liter, reabsorption of which of the following electrolytes increases proportionally?

   a. hydrogen

   b. potassium

   c. sodium

   d. bicarbonate

59. A patient is admitted with 1000 mL of diarrhea per day for the last 3 days. An IV of 0.45% NaCl mixed with 5% dextrose is infusing. Which of the following nursing interventions is the most appropriate?

   a. Get an infusion controller from central supply

   b. Mix all antibiotics in 0.45% NaCl with 5% dextrose.

   c. Check the patient's potassium level, and contact the doctor for IV additive orders.

   d. Assess the patient for signs of hyperkalemia.

60. Mrs. Jones is receiving digoxin and Lasix daily. Today, Mrs. Jones complains of nausea, and her apical pulse is 130 and irregular. Which of the following nursing interventions is the most appropriate?

   a. Hold the digoxin, and check the patient's potassium level.

   b. Remove the orange juice from the patient's tray.

   c. Identify the patient as high risk for hyperkalemia.

   d. Assess the patient for other signs of hypernatremia.

61. The type of fluid used to manipulate fluid shifts among compartments is:

   a. whole blood

   b. TPN

   c. albumin

   d. Ensure

62. Marathon runners are at high risk for fluid volume deficit. Which one of the following is a related factor?

   a. decreased diuresis

   b. disease-related processes

   c. decreased breathing and perspiration

   d. increased breathing and perspiration

63. A patient has a nursing diagnosis of fluid volume deficit. Which one of the following medications could potentially exacerbate the problem?

   a. Synthroid

   b. Digoxin

   c. Lasix

   d. Insulin

64. In renal regulation of water balance, the functions of angiotensin II include:

   a. blood clotting within the nephron

   b. increasing progesterone secretion into the renal tubules

   c. catalyzing calcium rich nutrients

   d. selectively constricting portions of the arteriole in the nephron

65. The majority of gastrointestinal reabsorption of water occurs in:

   a. the small intestines

   b. the esophagus

   c. the colon

   d. the stomach

66. Etiologies associated with hypomagnesemia include:

a. decreased vitamin D intake
b. constipation
c. malabsorption syndrome
d. renal failure

67. Magnesium performs all of the following functions *except:*
    a. contributing to vasoconstriction
    b. assisting in cardiac muscle contraction
    c. facilitating sodium transport
    d. assisting in protein metabolism

68. Magnesium reabsorption is controlled by:
    a. loop of Henle
    b. glomerulus
    c. pituitary
    d. parathyroid hormone

69. Symptoms of hypermagnesemia may include:
    a. hypertension
    b. tachycardia
    c. hyperactive deep-tendon reflexes
    d. cardiac arrhythmias

70. When teaching a patient about foods high in magnesium, the nurse would *not* include:
    a. green vegetables
    b. butter
    c. nuts
    d. fruit

71. Which of the following nursing diagnoses might apply to a patient with isotonic FVD?
    a. altered urinary elimination
    b. decreased cardiac output
    c. increased cardiac output
    d. ineffective airway clearance

72. Which of the following findings would the nurse expect to assess in a patient with hypotonic FVE?
    a. poor skin turgor and increased thirst
    b. weight gain and thirst
    c. interstitial edema and hypertension
    d. hypotension and pitting edema

73. Which of the following nursing diagnoses might apply to a patient with hypertonic FVE?

a. ineffective airway clearance
b. potential for decreased cardiac output
c. ineffective breathing pattern
d. potential for increased cardiac output

74. Isotonic FVD can result from:
    a. GI fluid loss through diarrhea
    b. insensible water loss during prolonged fever
    c. inadequate ingestion of fluids and electrolytes
    d. impaired thirst regulation

75. The danger of fluid sequestered in the third space is that the fluid:
    a. is hypertonic and can cause hypervolemia
    b. is hypotonic and can cause water intoxication
    c. is not available for circulation
    d. contains large amounts of acids

76. Which of the following clinical conditions exacerbates electrolyte excretion?
    a. nasogastric feedings
    b. use of surgical drains
    c. immobility from fractures
    d. chronic water drinking

77. Which of the following electrolytes are lost as a result of vomiting?
    a. bicarbonate and calcium
    b. sodium and hydrogen
    c. sodium and potassium
    d. hydrogen and potassium

78. Bicarbonate is lost during which of the following clinical conditions?
    a. diarrhea
    b. diuresis
    c. diaphoresis
    d. vomiting

79. Disease of which of the following structures is most likely to affects electrolyte reabsorption?
    a. glomerulus
    b. renal tubules
    c. bladder
    d. renal pelvis

80. The balance of anions to cations as it occurs across cell membranes is known as:

a. osmotic activity
b. electrical neutrality
c. electrical stability
d. sodium-potassium pump

81. Body fluids perform which of the following functions?
a. transport nutrients
b. transport electrical charges
c. cushion the organs
d. facilitate fat metabolism

82. The interstitial space holds approximately how many liters?
a. 3 liters
b. 6 liters
c. 9 liters
d. 12 liters

83. The intracellular compartment holds water and:
a. proteins
b. glucose
c. sodium
d. uric acid

84. The majority of the body's water is contained in which of the following fluid compartments?
a. intracellular
b. interstitial
c. intravascular
d. extracellular

85. The extracellular fluid space holds water, electrolytes, proteins and:
a. red blood cells
b. potassium
c. lipids
d. nucleic acids

86. A diet containing the minimum daily sodium requirement for an adult would be:
a. a no-salt-added diet
b. a diet including 2 gm sodium
c. a diet including 4 gm sodium
d. a 1500-calorie weight-loss diet

87. Sodium balance is important for which of the following functions?
a. transmitting impulses in nerve and muscle fibers via the calcium-potassium pump
b. exchanging for magnesium and attracting chloride

c. combining with hydrogen and chloride for acid–base balance
d. exchanging for potassium and attracting chloride

88. Sodium levels are affected by the secretion of which of the following hormones?
a. progesterone and aldosterone
b. ADH and ACTH
c. antidiuretic hormone and FSH
d. ECF and aldosterone

89. An 85-year-old patient with a feeding tube has been experiencing severe watery stool. The patient is lethargic and has poor skin turgor, a pulse of 120, and hyperactive reflexes. Nursing interventions would include:
a. measuring and recording intake and output and daily weights
b. administering salt tablets and monitoring hypertonic parenteral solutions
c. administering sedatives
d. applying wrist restraints to avoid displacement of the feeding tube

90. A patient with a diagnosis of bipolar disorder has been drinking copious amounts of water and voiding frequently. The patient is experiencing muscle cramps and twitching, and is reporting dizziness. The nurse checks lab work for:
a. complete blood count results, particularly the platelets
b. electrolytes, particularly the serum sodium
c. urine analysis, particularly for the presence of white blood cells
d. EEG results

91. When recording a patient's intake, the nurse would include:
a. 120 mL of juice, 1 cup of mashed potatoes, and 700 mL IV solution
b. 500 mL of tube feeding, 60 mL of lactulose by mouth, and 750 mL IV solution
c. 1 hamburger, 1/2 cup of carrots, and 1 cup of ice cream
d. 750 mL IV solution, 1 cup of ice

cream, and 1 cup of tapioca pudding

92. When assessing a patient's intake and output, the nurse would note the following abnormal findings:
   a. decreased urine output and the presence of edema
   b. weight gain and dyspnea
   c. rapid pulse and decreased urine output
   d. distended jugular vein and tachycardia

93. A cancer patient comes to the emergency department complaining of a high fever. The patient states "I've been sweating a lot, and I'm really thirsty." The nurse explains that:
   a. "Due to the fever, you have lost fluid by sweating and your body is trying to compensate by getting you to take in more fluids."
   b. "You're sweaty and thirsty because you have been really hot. It will pass when the fever is over."
   c. "Fever doesn't usually cause sweating and thirst. Has there been something else going on?"
   d. "This is just a side effect of your chemotherapy. When you finish your treatment, it will go away."

94. Which of the following medical problems would place a patient at risk for metabolic acidosis?
   a. retention of bicarbonate
   b. lactic acid deficit
   c. aspirin overdose
   d. constipation

95. Which of the following series of assessment findings indicate respiratory alkalosis?
   a. dizziness, an excited state, and flaccid muscles
   b. high serum potassium, flaccid muscles, and paresthesia
   c. low serum potassium, confusion, and paresthesia

   d. high serum chloride, low serum potassium, and dizziness

96. The nurse is caring for a patient with IV orders for lactated Ringer's solution to infuse at 100 mL per hour. When doing the first assessment, the nurse would:
   a. Check that the ordered solution is hanging and the flow rate is within 2 hours.
   b. Check the the ordered solution is hanging and the flow rate is accurate.
   c. Discontinue the infusion after 100 cc's have infused.
   d. Check the IV site only.

97. The nurse assesses a patient's IV site and finds that it is red, hot, and tender to touch. The most appropriate first action is:
   a. Stop the infusion and remove the IV.
   b. Apply a warm soak to the site and reevaluate.
   c. Stop the infusion and restart the IV in the same area.
   d. Call the physician to evaluate.

98. In a severe burn, which electrolyte shifts from the ECF to the ICF?
   a. sodium
   b. potassium
   c. magnesium
   d. chloride

99. Sodium and potassium levels are altered in cirrhosis because of the presence of:
   a. antidiuretic hormone (ADH)
   b. nitrogen
   c. aldosterone
   d. ammonia

100. In SIADH, water intake should be:
   a. encouraged
   b. restricted
   c. no change in water intake
   d. given intravenously

Answer Sheet for Comprehensive Test Questions

With a pencil, blacken the circle under the option you have chosen for your correct answer.

	A	B	C	D		A	B	C	D		A	B	C	D
1.	○	○	○	○	21.	○	○	○	○	41.	○	○	○	○
2.	○	○	○	○	22.	○	○	○	○	42.	○	○	○	○
3.	○	○	○	○	23.	○	○	○	○	43.	○	○	○	○
4.	○	○	○	○	24.	○	○	○	○	44.	○	○	○	○
5.	○	○	○	○	25.	○	○	○	○	45.	○	○	○	○
6.	○	○	○	○	26.	○	○	○	○	46.	○	○	○	○
7.	○	○	○	○	27.	○	○	○	○	47.	○	○	○	○
8.	○	○	○	○	28.	○	○	○	○	48.	○	○	○	○
9.	○	○	○	○	29.	○	○	○	○	49.	○	○	○	○
10.	○	○	○	○	30.	○	○	○	○	50.	○	○	○	○
11.	○	○	○	○	31.	○	○	○	○	51.	○	○	○	○
12.	○	○	○	○	32.	○	○	○	○	52.	○	○	○	○
13.	○	○	○	○	33.	○	○	○	○	53.	○	○	○	○
14.	○	○	○	○	34.	○	○	○	○	54.	○	○	○	○
15.	○	○	○	○	35.	○	○	○	○	55.	○	○	○	○
16.	○	○	○	○	36.	○	○	○	○	56.	○	○	○	○
17.	○	○	○	○	37.	○	○	○	○	57.	○	○	○	○
18.	○	○	○	○	38.	○	○	○	○	58.	○	○	○	○
19.	○	○	○	○	39.	○	○	○	○	59.	○	○	○	○
20.	○	○	○	○	40.	○	○	○	○	60.	○	○	○	○

Answer Sheet for Comprehensive Test Questions

	A	B	C	D		A	B	C	D		A	B	C	D
61.	○	○	○	○	75.	○	○	○	○	89.	○	○	○	○
62.	○	○	○	○	76.	○	○	○	○	90.	○	○	○	○
63.	○	○	○	○	77.	○	○	○	○	91.	○	○	○	○
64.	○	○	○	○	78.	○	○	○	○	92.	○	○	○	○
65.	○	○	○	○	79.	○	○	○	○	93.	○	○	○	○
66.	○	○	○	○	80.	○	○	○	○	94.	○	○	○	○
67.	○	○	○	○	81.	○	○	○	○	95.	○	○	○	○
68.	○	○	○	○	82.	○	○	○	○	96.	○	○	○	○
69.	○	○	○	○	83.	○	○	○	○	97.	○	○	○	○
70.	○	○	○	○	84.	○	○	○	○	98.	○	○	○	○
71.	○	○	○	○	85.	○	○	○	○	99.	○	○	○	○
72.	○	○	○	○	86.	○	○	○	○	100.	○	○	○	○
73.	○	○	○	○	87.	○	○	○	○					
74.	○	○	○	○	88.	○	○	○	○					

COMPREHENSIVE TEST ANSWER KEY

1. *Correct response: c*
Normal serum concentrations of chloride range from 95 to 208 mEq/L.
a. High chloride levels are above 108 mEq/L.
b. Low chloride levels are below 95 mEq/L.
d. A chloride level of 96 is on the low border of normal.
Knowledge/Physiologic/Assessment

2. *Correct response: b*
Diabetes is associated with decreased levels of serum chloride.
a, c, and d. Nephritis, eclampsia, and cardiac disease are associated with elevated levels of serum chloride.
Knowledge/Physiologic/Assessment

3. *Correct response: c*
Chloride is a major anion found in extracellular fluid.
a. A compound occurs when two ions are bound together.
b. Chloride is an ion, but this is too general an answer.
d. HCO_3 is a cation.
Knowledge/Physiologic/NA

4. *Correct response: a*
Administration of phosphate binders (Amphojel and Basajel) will reduce the serum phosphate levels.
b, c, and d. Fleet's phospho-soda, milk, and vitamin D will increase serum phosphate levels.
Application/Safe care/Implementation

5. *Correct response: c*
Metastatic bone lesions are associated with hypercalcemia caused by accelerated bone metabolism and release of calcium into the serum.
a, b, and d. Renal failure, inadequate calcium intake, and vitamin D deficiency may cause hypocalcemia.
Comprehension/Safe care/Assessment

6. *Correct response: d*
Urinary calculi may occur with hypercalcemia.
a. Shortened, not prolonged, QRS complex would be seen in hypercalcemia.
b and c. Tetany and petechiae are signs of hypocalcemia.
Comprehension/Safe care/Assessment

7. *Correct response: b*
Calcium gluconate is used for replacement in deficiency states.
a and c. Calcitonin and loop diuretics are administered to lower serum calcium.
d. Ambulation is recommended to prevent the movement of calcium from the bone.
Comprehension/Safe care/Implementation

8. *Correct response: d*
Renal failure can reduce magnesium excretion, leading to hypermagnesemia.
a. Diabetic ketoacidosis, not insulin shock, is a cause of hypermagnesemia.
b. Hypoadrenalism, not hyperadrenalism, is a cause of hypermagnesemia.
c. Nausea and vomiting lead to hypomagnesemia.
Application/Safe care/Analysis

9. *Correct response: b*
In a patient with hypermagnesemia, administration of calcium gluconate will antagonize the cardiac effects of magnesium.
a. Although calcium gluconate will raise serum calcium levels, that is not the purpose for its administration.
c and d. Calcium gluconate does not lower calcium or magnesium levels.
Application/Safe care/Implementation

10. *Correct response: b*

In hypomagnesemia, a patient on digoxin is likely to develop digitalis toxicity.

a and c. Neither of these medications has toxicity as a side effect.

d. CAPD is not a medication.

Analysis/Safe care/Evaluation

11. *Correct response: c*

Osmotic pressure is the phenomenon that causes fluids to move in both directions simultaneously; it is not a parameter that is assessed.

a, b, and d. Skin turgor; intake and output; and blood pressure, pulse, and central venous pressure are physical assessment parameters the nurse would consider when assessing fluid and electrolyte balance.

Application/Safe care/Assessment

12. *Correct response: d*

Perspiration and the fluid lost via the lungs are termed insensible losses; normally, insensible losses equal about 1000 mL/day.

a, b, and c. These types of fluid losses are measurable and therefore are *not* insensible.

Knowledge/Physiologic/NA

13. *Correct response: b*

When hyponatremia is severe, hypertonic solutions may be used but should be infused with caution due to the potential for development of CHF.

a and c. In SIADH, hypotonic and isotonic solutions are not indicated because urine output is minimal, so water is retained. This water retention dilutes serum sodium levels, making the patient hyponatremic and necessitating administration of hypertonic solutions to balance sodium and water.

d. Normotonic solutions do not exist.

Application/

14. *Correct response: a*

Aldosterone is secreted in response to fluid loss. Aldosterone causes sodium reabsorption and potassium elimination, further exacerbating hypokalemia.

b, c, and d. Hyperkalemia, hyponatremia, and hypernatremia do not result from aldosterone secretion.

Comprehension/Physiologic/Analysis

15. *Correct response: c*

Poor skin turgor is a sign of dehydration, not fluid overload.

a, b, and d. Bounding pulse, bulging neck veins, and rales are symptoms observed in patients with fluid overload.

Comprehension/Safe care/Assessment

16. *Correct response: b*

Potassium must be well diluted and given slowly because rapid administration will cause cardiac arrest.

a, c, and d. Potassium must *never* be administered rapidly as a bolus because cardiac arrest will result.

Application/Safe care/Implementation

17. *Correct response: d*

Hyporeflexia is a symptom of hypokalemia.

a, b, and c. Hypotension, pH above 7.45, and hyperglycemia are symptoms of hypokalemia.

Comprehension/ Safe Care/Assessment

18. *Correct response: b*

Oral potassium supplements are known to irritate gastrointestinal (GI) mucosa and should be diluted.

a, c, and d. When taken undiluted, on an empty stomach, or at bedtime (when the stomach is empty), oral potassium supplements will cause GI irritation.

Knowledge/Safe care/Implementation

19. *Correct response: b*

Normal venous blood pH ranges from 7.31 to 7.41.

a and d. These are not normal pH values.

c. Normal arterial blood pH ranges from 7.35 to 7.45.

Knowledge/Safe care/Assessment

20. *Correct response: d*
Respiratory regulation of acid–base balance involves the elimination or retention of carbon dioxide.
a, b, and c. Oxygen, hydrogen, and hydroxide are not involved in the respiratory regulation of acid–base balance.
Knowledge/Physiologic/NA

21. *Correct response: d*
Pulse oximetry yields oxygen saturation levels, which is not a measure of acid–base balance.
a and b. Respiratory regulation of acid–base balance involves the retention or elimination of carbon dioxide through adjustments in the rate and depth of respirations.
c. Arterial blood gases will indicate CO_2 levels.
Application/Safe care/Assessment

22. *Correct response: b*
Isotonic FVD involves an equal decrease in solute concentration and water volume.
a, c, and d. These conditions produce different changes in the solute concentration and water volume.
Comprehension/Safe care/Analysis

23. *Correct response: b*
Weight loss of more than 0.50 lb. is considered to be fluid loss.
a. Weight loss of 0.25 lb is not significant enough to be considered fluid loss.
c and d. Although 1 lb. and 1 kg could be considered fluid loss, the nurse would begin to identify fluid loss with a weight loss of 0.50 lb.
Application/Safe care/Assessment

24. *Correct response: b*
Hypotonic fluid volume excess (FVE) involves an increase in water volume without an increase in sodium concentration. Increased sodium intake is part of the management of this condition.

a. Decreased sodium intake will exacerbate the condition, since hypotonic FVE is associated with low sodium.
c. Fluids are restricted, not increased.
d. Intake of potassium-rich foods is not related to hypotonic FVE.
Application/Health promotion/Implementation

25. *Correct response: b*
In diffusion, the solute moves from an area of higher concentration to one of lower concentration, creating osmotic pressure.
a. Osmotic pressure is related to the process of osmosis.
c. Filtration is created by hydrostatic pressure.
d. Capillary dynamics are related to fluid exchange at the intravascular and interstitial levels.
Knowledge/Physiologic/NA

26. *Correct response: d*
Arterial baroreceptors and stretch receptors help maintain fluid balance by increasing urine output in response to a rise in arterial pressure.
a and b. Decreased or increased sodium reabsorption occurs in response to the secretion of the atrial natriuretic factor.
c. Increased, not decreased urine output occurs.
Knowledge/Physiologic/Analysis

27. *Correct response: c*
Normal serum sodium level ranges from 136 to 145 mEq/L.
a, b, and d. These are not normal sodium levels.
Knowledge/Health promotion/Assessment

28. *Correct response: d*
Water loss will not lead to hyponatremia.
a, b, and c. Water gain, diuretic therapy, and diaphoresis are etiologies of hyponatremia.
Application/Health promotion/Assessment

29. *Correct response: c*

Hyponatremia involves a decreased concentration of sodium in relation to fluid volume, so restricting fluid intake is indicated.

a. Hypotonic fluids will exacerbate hyponatremia.

b. Fluids are restricted, not encouraged.

d. Sodium intake is restricted, not encouraged.

Application/Safe care/Implementation

30. *Correct response: b*

Alkalosis is indicated by a pH above 7.45.

a. Acidosis is indicated by a pH below 7.35.

c. Homeostasis is present when a normal pH is present.

d. Neutrality is the pH range from 7.35 to 7.45.

Application/Safe care/Assessment

31. *Correct response: c*

Osmosis is defined as the diffusion of water through a semipermeable membrane to a solution with a lower concentration of water.

a. Filtration is the process in which fluids are pushed through biologic membranes by unequal processes.

b and d. Diffusion (brownian motion) is the random kinetic motion causing atoms and molecules to spread out evenly.

Knowledge/Physiologic/NA

32. *Correct response: d*

A patient's sex does not influence the percentage of total body water.

a, b, and c. A patient's age and amount of fat tissue and lean muscle do influence the percentage of total body water.

Knowledge/Health promotion/Assessment

33. *Correct response: c*

Tachycardia, poor tissue turgor, and hypotension are symptoms of FVD.

a, b, and d. Rales, bounding pulse, and bulging neck veins are symptoms of FVE.

Application/Safe care/Assessment

34. *Correct response: a*

Water intoxication is a potential complication associated with hypotonic fluid administration.

b, c, and d. FVE, cellular dehydration, and cell shrinkage are potential complications of hypertonic fluid administration.

Application/Safe care/Implementation

35. *Correct response: c*

A solution of 0.9% saline is isotonic.

a, b, and d. Solutions of 0.33% and 0.45% saline and D5W are hypotonic (e.g., osmolar concentration is lower than plasma).

Knowledge/Safe care/Implementation

36. *Correct response: a*

Uncompensated metabolic alkalosis is indicated by ABG values of pH 7.48, $PaCO_2$ 42, and HCO_3 30.

b. These ABG values indicate metabolic alkalosis, partially compensated.

c. These ABG values indicate respiratory alkalosis, partially compensated.

d. These ABG values indicate respiratory alkalosis, uncompensated.

Comprehension/Safe care/Analysis

37. *Correct response: b*

The body attempts to compensate for metabolic alkalosis by decreasing the respiratory rate and conserving carbon dioxide (an acid).

a. This response is incorrect.

c and d. Urine volume does not influence acid–base balance.

Analysis/Physiologic/Assessment

38. *Correct response: b*

A decreased respiratory rate is a symptom of metabolic acidosis and may be caused by the body's attempt to compensate for the metabolic alkalosis.

a, c, and d. Decreased serum potassium, paresthesias, and stupor are common symptoms of metabolic alkalosis.

Comprehension/Safe care/Assessment

39. *Correct response: c*
Platelets and cryoprecipitate can be infused quickly.
a and b. PRBC and FFP should be administered over 1 1/2 to 4 hours.
d. Dextran is not a blood product.
Application/Safe care/Implementation

40. *Correct response: a*
Hypotonic solutions provide free water, which helps the kidneys eliminate solute.
b. Hypotonic solutions are poor sources of sodium and chloride ions.
c. Excessive volumes are not recommended in early postoperative periods since stress can increase ADH secretion.
d. Hypertonic solutions are used to treat hyponatremia.
Comprehension/Safe care/ Implementation

41. *Correct response: c*
An increase in body temperature indicates a possible transfusion reaction and requires immediate discontinuation of the infusion.
b. There is inadequate evidence for sepsis to be considered.
a and d. An elevated body temperature is neither a normal nor an expected finding.
Analysis/Safe care/Analysis

42. *Correct response: d*
ACTH stimulates release of aldosterone, which in turn acts on the tubules to reabsorb sodium. When this occurs, the cation potassium is excreted.
a and b. Chloride is not involved in this process.
c. Potassium reabsorption is not influenced by the endocrine system.
Comprehension/Physiologic/Planning

43. *Correct response: a*
Phosphorus is the chief anion found in the ICF.
c and b. Potassium and sodium are cations.

d. Chloride is the chief anion found in the ECF.
Knowledge/Physiologic/Assessment

44. *Correct response: a*
Potassium is the major ICF cation.
b. sodium is the major ECF cation
c. Phosphorus is the major ICF anion.
d. Magnesium is the second-most abundant cation in the ICF.
Knowledge/Physiological/Assessment

45. *Correct response: d*
Hypophosphatemia may occur secondary to alcoholism.
a and c. Liver cirrhosis and Paget's disease generally have no effect on phosphorous levels.
b. Renal failure is usually associated with hyperphosphatemia.
Knowledge/Physiologic/Assessment

46. *Correct response: c*
Because calcium and phosphorus ratios are inversely proportional, when phosphorous levels are high, calcium levels are low.
a, b, and d. These condition have no influence on phosphorus levels.
Comprehension/Safe care/Analysis

47. *Correct response: c*
Some calcium is bound to protein, so abnormal calcium levels are analyzed in relation to proteins.
a, b, and d. Sodium, glucose, and fats are not related to calcium levels.
Knowledge/Physiological/Analysis

48. *Correct response: a*
Calcium is absorbed in the GI tract under the influence of vitamin D in its biologically active form.
b, c, and d. Calcium reabsorption is not related to these elements in any way.
Knowledge/Physiologic/Analysis

49. *Correct response: b*
A patient with hypocalcemia may bleed, since calcium is required for normal blood clotting.

a and d. These nursing diagnoses are appropriate for a patient with hypercalcemia.

c. Ineffective airway clearing is not associated with fluctuating calcium levels.

Application/Safe care/Analysis (Dx)

50. *Correct response: d*
When calcium levels rise, calcitonin is secreted from the thyroid; this hormone moves calcium from plasma into bone.

a and b. These hormones are not secreted in response to calcium levels.

c. Parathyroid hormone is secreted in response to lowered calcium levels; this hormone moves calcium from bone into plasma.

Knowledge/Physiologic/Analysis

51. *Correct response: c*
The presence of hydrogen ions determines a solution's acidity.

a, b, and d. These ions do not influence a solution's acidity or alkalinity.

Knowledge/Physiologic/Assessment

52. *Correct response: c*
The lungs use carbon dioxide to regulate hydrogen ion concentration.

a, b, and d. These are not actions that the lungs perform.

Comprehension/Physiologic/NA

53. *Correct response: b*
Through changes in the rate and depth of respirations, acid–base balance is achieved via CO_2 elimination and retention.

a. Mucus production is not part of the pulmonary regulatory system.

c and d. These responses refer to ways in which the kidneys balance acids and bases.

Knowledge/Physiologic/Assessment

54. *Correct response: a*
The gases measured by ABGs are oxygen and carbon dioxide.

b, c, and d. Bicarbonate and hydro-

gen are ions; their ratio is measured in the pH.

Comprehension/Physiologic/Assessment

55. *Correct response: a*
To maintain acid–base balance, chloride shifts into and out of red blood cells in exchange for bicarbonate.

b and c. Although these are roles of chloride, they do not help balance acids and bases.

d. Chloride does not act to separate carbonic acid.

Knowledge/Physiologic/Assessment

56. *Correct response: d*
Chloride reabsorption depends on sodium reabsorption, which is regulated by aldosterone in the distal tubule and collecting ducts.

a, b, and c. These hormones do not effect chloride reabsorption.

Knowledge/Physiologic/Assessment

57. *Correct response: b*
Chloride is absorbed in the bowel, mainly the duodenum and jejunum.

a. Chloride absorption does not take place in the stomach.

c and d. Chloride reabsorption does not take place in the liver and kidney.

Knowledge/Physiologic/NA

58. *Correct response: d*
When chloride concentrations drop below 95 mEq/liter, bicarbonate reabsorption increased proportionally, causing metabolic alkalosis.

a, b, and c. These are cations, chloride is an anion; a cation must always exchange for a cation in order to maintain electrical neutrality.

Comprehension/Safe care/Analysis

59. *Correct response: c*
Potassium is lost via the GI and renal systems. Prolonged or excessive diarrhea can lead to hypokalemia. In the event of hypokalemia, a potassium additive would likely be prescribed.

a. There is no information to indicate the need for this safety measure.

b. Antibiotics should be mixed in the appropriate solution; the patient situation provides no information indicating this action.

d. There is no information indicating hyperkalemia.

Application/Physiologic/Implementation

60. Correct response: a
Patients experiencing hypokalemia are at risk for digitalis toxicity. Nausea and irregular pulse are signs of digitalis toxicity.

b and c. These refer to concerns regarding hyperkalemia.

d. Hypernatremia is not associated with digitalis toxicity.

Analysis/Safe care/Implementation

61. Correct response: c
Albumin is a colloid that is used to manipulate fluid shifts among compartments.

a. Whole blood is used to replace blood volume.

b. TPN is used for patients who are unable to take in food or fluid.

d. Ensure is high caloric nutritional supplement; it is not used to manipulate fluid shifts.

Comprehension/Physiologic/Planning

62. Correct response: d
Excessive fluid can be lost if breathing and perspiration are at an increased rate for a prolonged period.

a. This is not related to fluid loss.

b. This response is incorrect.

c. This is not an etiology for fluid loss.

Application/Physiologic/Analysis

63. Correct response: c
Lasix will contribute to fluid loss through its action as a diuretic.

a, b, and d. Synthroid (a synthetic thyroid replacement), digoxin (a cardiotonic glycoside), and insulin (a hormone) would not exacerbate fluid volume deficit.

Comprehension/Safe care/Assessment

64. Correct response: d
As part of the renal regulation of

water balance, angiotensin II selectively constricts portions of the arteriole in the nephron.

a, b, and c. These responses do not refer to angiotensin II or any functions of renal regulation.

Knowledge/Physiologic/Analysis

65. Correct response: a
Approximately 85% to 95% of water absorption takes place in the small intestines. The colon absorbs only 500 to 1000 mL.

b, c, and d. These responses are incorrect.

Knowledge/Physiologic/Assessment

66. Correct response: c
Malabsorption syndrome is associated with hypomagnesemia.

a and b. Increased vitamin D intake and diarrhea are associated with hypomagnesemia.

d. This response is incorrect.

Knowledge/Physiologic/Assessment

67. Correct response: a
Magnesium contributes to vasodilation, not vasoconstriction.

a, c, and d. These are all functions of magnesium.

Knowledge/Safe care/NA

68. Correct response: a
The Loop of Henle is responsible for magnesium reabsorption.

b, c, and d. These responses are incorrect.

Knowledge/Physiologic/NA

69. Correct response: d
Cardiac arrhythmias are associated with hypermagnesemia.

a, b, and c. Hypertension, tachycardia, and hyperactive reflexes are signs of hypomagnesemia.

Knowledge/Safe care/Assessment

70. Correct response: b
Butter is not high in magnesium.

a, c, and d. These foods are good sources of magnesium.

Knowledge/Safe care/Implementation

71. Correct response: b
Decreased cardiac output is a nursing diagnosis associated with isotonic FVD. Other appropriate nursing diagnoses include altered tissue perfusion, potential for injury, and ineffective breathing pattern.
a, c, and d. These diagnoses are not associated with FVD.
Application/Safe care/Analysis (Dx)

72. Correct response: b
Weight gain and thirst are symptoms of hypotonic FVE; other symptoms include excretion of dilute urine, non-pitting edema, dysrhythmias, and hyponatremia.
a and d. Poor skin turgor, thirst, hypotension, and pitting edema are signs of hypertonic FVD.
c. Interstitial edema and hypertension are signs of isotonic FVE.
Application/Safe care/Assessment

73. Correct response: b
Potential for decreased cardiac output is a nursing diagnosis associated with hypertonic FVE.
a, c, and d. These nursing diagnoses are not applicable to hypertonic FVE.
Application/Safe care/Analysis (Dx)

74. Correct response: c
Isotonic FVD may result from inadequate intake of fluids and electrolytes that can occur secondary to an inability to ingest orally.
a. GI fluid loss through diarrhea is an etiology of hypotonic FVD.
b. Insensible water loss during prolonged fever is a cause of hypertonic FVD.
d. Impaired thirst regulation is a cause of hypertonic FVD.
Application/Safe care/Analysis

75. Correct response: c
In third-spacing, fluid is sequestered and is unavailable to the general circulation.
a, c, and d. These responses have no relationship to the third spacing of fluids.
Comprehension/Safe care/Analysis

76. Correct response: b
Surgical drains will cause a fluid loss, and electrolytes are eliminated along with the fluid.
a. Nasogastric feedings are a source of electrolyte intake, not elimination.
c. Immobility does not cause electrolytes to be eliminated.
d. Chronic water drinking will change electrolyte levels as a result of dilution, but it does not contribute in any way to electrolyte excretion.
Analysis/Safe care/Evaluation

77. Correct response: d
In upper gastrointestinal fluid loss, hydrogen and potassium are lost because these electrolytes are present in abundance in the stomach.
a, b, and c. These responses are incorrect because bicarbonate, calcium, and sodium are not abundantly present.
Comprehension/Physiologic/Assessment

78. Correct answer: a
Bicarbonate is lost in diarrhea because the lower intestinal tract contains fluids rich in bicarbonate.
b. Diuresis is excessive urination that tends to cause a loss of sodium, potassium, and chloride.
c. Diaphoresis is excessive sweating that tends to cause a loss of sodium and chloride.
d. Vomiting tends to cause a loss of potassium and hydrogen.
Comprehension/Physiologic/Assessment

79. Correct response: b
The renal tubules are the site of electrolyte reabsorption.
a. The glomerulus is the site of electrolyte filtration.
c. The bladder is where urine is stored.
d. The renal pelvis is where urine

travels as it moves from the collecting ducts to the ureter.
Knowledge/Physiologic/Assessment

80. *Correct response: b*
Electrical neutrality refers to a state in which the same number of positively charged ions and negatively charged ions are present on either side of the membrane.
    a. Osmotic activity refers to the attraction of a solute to a solvent.
    c. There is no such concept as electrical stability in electrolyte balance.
    d. Sodium-potassium pump refers to the exchange of electrolytes.
Knowledge/Physiologic/Assessment

81. *Correct answer: a*
Body fluids facilitate the transport of nutrients, hormones, proteins, and other molecules.
    b. Electrical charges are not transported.
    c and d. These responses are incorrect.
Knowledge/Physiologic/Assessment

82. *Correct response: c*
The interstitial space holds 9 liters.
    b, c, and d. No fluid compartment holds these amounts of fluid.
Knowledge/Physiologic/Assessment

83. *Correct response: a*
The intracellular compartment holds large amounts of water and proteins. Potassium, lipids, and nucleic acids are also components of the intracellular compartment.
    b, c, d. These are not components of the intracellular compartment.
Knowledge/Physiologic/Assessment

84. *Correct response: a*
The intracellular compartment holds two thirds of total body water.
    b, c, and d. The extracellular compartment is the interstitial space *plus* the intravascular space. The extracellular compartment accounts for one third of total body water.
Knowledge/Physiologic/Assessment

85. *Correct response: a*
The extracellular space contains red blood cells, white blood cells, and platelets in addition to water, electrolytes, and proteins.
    b, c, and d. Potassium, lipids, and nucleic acids are intracellular components.
Knowledge/Physiologic/Assessment

86. *Correct response: b*
The minimum sodium requirement for adults is 2 gm daily. Most adults consume more than this because sodium is abundant in almost all foods.
    a. This response is incorrect.
    c. 4 gm daily would be too high.
    d. A 1500-calorie weight-loss diet does not give information regarding the salt content.
Knowledge/Health promotion/Planning

87. *Correct response: d*
Sodium influences the levels of potassium and chloride by exchanging for potassium and attracting chloride.
    a. Sodium balance facilitates impulse transmission by participating in the sodium-potassium pump.
    b. Magnesium is not involved in the exchange or attraction.
    c. Acid–base balance involves sodium combining with bicarbonate and chloride.
Knowledge/Physiologic/Assessment

88. *Correct response: b*
The endocrine system secretes aldosterone and ADH to help regulate sodium levels. The pituitary secretes adrenocorticotropin hormone to help regulate sodium.
    a and c. These are reproductive hormones.
    d. ECF is not a hormone; it is the abbreviation for extracellular fluid.
Knowledge/Physiologic/Assessment

89. *Correct response: a*
The patient is exhibiting signs of hypernatremia and dehydration. The most appropriate nursing intervention

is to measure and record intake and output and daily weight.

b. Administration of sodium tablets is not part of the treatment for hypernatremia. Also, the nurse would expect that the IV solutions used for hypernatremia would be hypotonic.

c and d. There are no clinical indications for these measures.

Analysis/Safe care/Implementation

90. *Correct response: B*
The patient is exhibiting behavior that could lead to a sodium and water imbalance and is exhibiting signs of hyponatremia. The nurse would check the electrolytes with attention to the sodium level.

a and c. These laboratory results which are not related to the potential problem.

d. EEG (electroencephalogram) is a diagnostic test.

Application/Safe care/Assessment

91. *Correct response: b*
When recording a patient's intake, the nurse would include all fluids taken by mouth, by nasogastric route, or intravenously. Foods high in fluid content would be included.

a. This response is incorrect because it includes mashed potatoes

c. This response is incorrect because it includes the hamburger and carrots

d. This response is incorrect because it includes the pudding.

Comprehension/Safe care/ Implementation

92. *Correct response: a*
a. These are altered findings related to intake and output.

b, c, and d. These abnormal findings are related to assessment areas other than intake and output.

Comprehension/Safe care/Assessment

93. *Correct response: a*
Temperature elevation results in increased fluid loss through the skin.

b. This response indicates that the

fever may be associated with the other symptoms, but it does not provide correct information.

c and d. These responses are incorrect.

Analysis/Health promotion/ Implementation

94. *Correct response: c*
Metabolic acidosis is an acid–base imbalance caused by an increase in metabolic acids. In states in which metabolic acid buildup occurs, metabolic acidosis may occur. Salicylate toxicity causes a buildup of acids, causing metabolic acidosis; aspirin contains salicylate.

a and b. These responses indicate that acids are not accumulating.

d. Diarrhea causes a loss of bicarbonate through the GI system.

Comprehension/Physiologic/Assessment

95. *Correct response: c*
Apathy, tetany, carpopedal spasm, low serum potassium, low serum chloride, dizziness, and paresthesia are all assessment findings indicating respiratory alkalosis.

a, b, and d. These responses include some symptoms or laboratory data that are opposite the findings seen in respiratory alkalosis.

Knowledge/Safe care/Assessment

96. *Correct response: b*
When monitoring IV therapy, it is important that the nurse ensure that the right solution is infusing at the prescribed rate.

a. This response is incorrect.

c. This response does not reflect the IV orders.

d. Checking the IV site is only one aspect of the required assessment.

Application/Safe care/Assessment

97. *Correct response: a*
Stopping the infusion and removing the IV are actions taken for both local and systemic complications.

b and c. These are not appropriate actions.

d. Calling the physician may be appropriate depending on the situation, but not as a first action.

Analysis/Safe care/Implementation

98. *Correct answer: b*

Initially after a burn, intracellular potassium is released as cells are destroyed. After 4 to 5 days, potassium may shift from the ECF to the ICF.

a, c, and d. All electrolytes are affected by burns, but potassium shifts represent the most severe.

Comprehension/Physiologic/Assessment

99. *Correct answer: c*

In cirrhosis, aldosterone, as well as other hormones, are not metabolized. The presence of aldosterone leads to increased sodium reabsorption and subsequent potassium elimination.

a, b, and d. These choices do not affect sodium and potassium.

Comprehension/Physiologic/Assessment

100. *Correct answer: b*

In SIADH, the antidiuretic hormone is present in excess amounts. This causes too much water reabsorption, diluting the patient's serum. Water must then be restricted to avoid water intoxication.

a, c, and d. These are not appropriate interventions regarding fluid intake.

Application/Safe care/Intervention

Index

Note: Page numbers in *italics* indicate illustrations; those followed by d indicate display material; those followed by t indicate tables.